Manfred J. Poggel

# Parkinson´s disease

Manfred J. Poggel

# Parkinson´s disease

## How I was healed without chemicals

JustFiction Edition

Publisher:
JustFiction! Edition
is a trademark of
Dodo Books Indian Ocean Ltd., member of the OmniScriptum S.R.L Publishing group
str. A.Russo 15, of. 61, Chisinau-2068, Republic of Moldova Europe
Printed at: see last page
**ISBN: 978-620-3-57568-2**

# Parkinson's disease

*This book is dedicated, with my thanks and love,
to my wonderful wife, who carried me through
this difficult time and still carries me today.*

**Own Publishing House**

S. E. M.

Renate Poggel-Zündorf und Manfred J.Poggel

Author's note:

I have compiled the information in this book to the best of my knowledge and belief. I have used most of the treatments described myself and the reports on my experiences are based on this. Where I have not used a treatment which is described myself, I have made this clear. However, I cannot entirely rule out the possibility that I may have made one or two mistakes in the information which may become apparent over time.

The author and publisher accept no liability regarding the application of the treatments or medications described. The author does not provide any medical advice on treatments or medications; the statements in the book are the author's personal opinions. The applications described are not a replacement for medical treatment. The purpose of this book is exclusively to present various personal experiments which have been clearly successful. No promise of healing or recovery is made.

If you have a serious illness and/or long-term medical complaints you must consult a doctor or alternative practitioner. The author and publisher accept no liability for the accuracy of the statements made, their effects or interpretations from the text. Where registration details of trademarks or brand names are not explicitly specified, this does not necessarily mean that the name of the product is not protected. No liability for errors or omissions is accepted. The author and publisher do not intend to provide any form of medical or professional services.

Should the treatments I have discovered or my opinions on research into the causes of the disease appear sensible and useful to you, I would be grateful if you were to discuss them with your doctor or alternative practitioner and, if applicable, your health insurance provider.

# Manfred J. Poggel

# Parkinson's disease

How I was healed without chemicals

# Contents

## 'He who is ill long enough becomes a doctor himself'

… says a Chinese proverb. Left to conventional medicine, which does not investigate causes but merely treats symptoms, patients suffering from illnesses such as Parkinson's disease will remain 'incurable'.
It is time for this way of thinking to change.

What causes Parkinson's disease?
Ask your doctor! Be persistent. Do not let yourself be fobbed off. Be sceptical and question the answers you are given. Get at least one second opinion. I, in any case, have sometimes heard some rather adventurous explanations which I will describe here.
You are always told, 'You must take your tablets at the right time. After all, you have a chronic illness. You have Parkinson's disease; it's incurable. We'll do everything we can for you to slow down the disease for a few more years. You must bear in mind that you'll be in a wheelchair in five years.' After hearing these statements, it is no wonder that I was afraid.
The doctors who had treated me years before I was diagnosed with Parkinson's disease were truly sympathetic and compassionate. Yet I also felt a real sense of their helplessness as they could not cure this disease. They clearly simply did not know of any alternatives to their chemical preparations.

So it was that I found myself subjected to a marathon of expert assessments that went on for years. It reached its peak when a judge tried to have me sent to a clinic for psychiatric and pharmacological treatment. However, luckily for me, a chance suggestion from a physiotherapist awoke a determination in me to finally decline the pharmaceutical industry's chemical medications.

Nevertheless, it was clear to me that I would not be able to go down this path alone. Furthermore, I had no medical training. Simply understanding the vocabulary was a challenge for me at first. In my desperation, I asked the man upstairs for his help.
And it was granted.
I then began investigating the cause of my Parkinson's disease. And I found it. After I had discovered the cause, I obtained a wide range of information from naturopathic doctors and alternative practitioners which I have detailed here – treatments that I have tested myself with success.
Over the years, all of the information about treatments for and the possible causes of Parkinson's disease brought me to the knowledge which led me to write this book. Consequently, I present to you here the knowledge from my own new life *without* toxins. Meditation and spiritual guidance helped me, with time, to develop an understanding and knowledge in order to deal with my illness better and in a more relaxed way – and eventually also led me to recovery.
The first small successes already made me speechless and thankful. Of course, there were setbacks too, but the bad days became fewer and more far between as the years passed.

Today I can describe myself as cured. I have not been inside a doctor's surgery for three years. Not only that but my new basic lifestyle, the change in diet, the regular detoxification of heavy metals, fungi and viruses, and the other changes I have made have not only cured me of Parkinson's but have also made the rheumatic illnesses I have had since childhood, such as chronic polyarthritis, fibromyalgia and the beginnings of arthrosis in my knees, as well as headaches and the ulcer on the lower part of my left leg, disappear completely.

Therefore, with this book, I would like to give you the courage to view your 'fate' from the perspective of the possibilities of recovery. Above all, however, I would like to encourage you not to be afraid any longer. I discovered the real causes of my disease – by chance, through my own experience, and by talking to people with the same fate.

1. A person with a disease must be understood as a whole.
2. Illness is a lack of energy (vibrations).
3. There are no coincidences; we are controlled and guided.
4. Do not ask 'why me?' but 'why this?'.
5. Open yourself up to the natural possibilities of medicine.
6. Spiritual and physical activities heal us.
7. Spiritual experiences want to be implemented and used.
8. A healthy diet heals.
9. Trust in the healing powers within us.
10. Expand your awareness through new points of view.

The dreaded diagnosis of an 'incurable disease' awoke a fighting spirit in me and led me down the path of putting the healing process into action by investigating the cause, with energy transfers, with the power of the mind, and with the possibilities of natural medicine without harmful side effects, and motivated me to see it through to the end. This is a path that can give others hope, of that I am certain! Conventional medical practitioners like to refer to this as a spontaneous recovery. To this I say, 'No one else has succeeded in curing themselves. Healing is a blessing which comes from God.' And as every human being possesses these God-given powers of healing, what needs to be done is to activate them. This book will provide suggestions and help to all those who are affected by Parkinson's disease and all therapists.

I wish you all the best and hope that you understand my thoughts and suggestions as they are intended. I do not want to teach you; I want to offer you help to help yourself. I invite you to use my experience of a healthy lifestyle *without* chemicals for yourself, so that one day you will be able to enjoy a healthy day once again!


## Parkinson's – an incurable lifestyle disease?

Before I share with you my very personal life experiences and experiences with the disease, I would like to explain why I am doing so.

My observations and encounters over many years have shown me that there are a wide range of parallels in Parkinson's sufferers. These may be events which occurred before birth, such as the mother's fears or a premature birth, but also the sufferer's own experiences of serious cases of the flu or infections, cervical spine disorders, rheumatic diseases, viral diseases, depression, REM sleep behaviour disorders, ADD or ADHD, problems with the sense of smell, liver disease, all kinds of stress, unhealthy lifestyles, toxification and other factors. (In this context births by Caesarean section are also considered premature births if carried out more than three days before the due date.)
It is also interesting that Parkinson's disease occurs in a large number of people who have been self-employed or have worked in management positions and therefore been exposed to high levels of stress. According to Professor Volker Fintelmann, there is often a mental block (see part II, 26, Anthroposophic therapy) to overcoming these kinds of stresses.

In 1998, a particular gene was discovered during research at the Institute of Tropical Diseases in Hamburg. It sits on the short arm of chromosome 2 and has since been regarded as a significant trigger of Parkinson's disease in certain predisposed families. However, it is not this simple, as Parkinson's is also diagnosed in people who do not have this gene.

As is common knowledge, put in simple terms, a reduction in the messenger substance dopamine in the brain is considered to be the cause of Parkinson's disease. When Parkinson's is diagnosed, the level of dopamine in the then markedly light substantia nigra in the brain has already decreased by 90 percent. If not enough dopamine is or can be produced, this naturally leads to a lack of dopamine. But why is this? Why does conventional medicine not seem to be really and truly interested in the causes of this disease?

In 1817, the English doctor and pharmacist James Parkinson (1755–1824) described the symptoms of Parkinson's disease, making reference to ancient descriptions made by the Roman doctor Galen (129–199 AD). We find records of these symptoms as far back as around 1500 BC in Ayurvedic scripts. Erasistratus, a doctor in ancient Greece, also documented similar disease characteristics back in the third century BC. In the twelfth century AD, Saint Hildegard of Bingen described the 'shaking palsy'. It was not until the seventeenth century that Sylvius de la Boe made the distinction between the various forms of tremor.

James Parkinson believed that a cervical spine disorder was the cause of these symptoms. In 1884, the neurologist Professor Jean Martin Charcot was the first person to use the term 'Parkinson's disease'.

The changes in the black substance in the brain (the substantia nigra) were discovered by the doctor Konstantin N. Tretiakoff (1892–1958) in 1919. Since the 1940s, the area of the brain that is affected has been determined more exactly, and as of 1960 there has been a synthetic form of dopamine, known as L-dopa, which, due to the discoveries of Ehringer and Oleh Hornykiewicz, has opened up new methods of

treating Parkinson's disease. The dopamine replacement developed by Birkmayer and Barbeau represented the beginning of modern Parkinson's medication.
However, that is now 50 years ago and incidences of the disease have increased rapidly.

Other than dopamine replacements and antidepressants with severe side effects, I was not prescribed any other forms of modern medication. Clearly not much progress has been made in conventional medicine in the past few decades when it comes to Parkinson's disease. Even the urgently necessary physiotherapy was only prescribed to me after I explicitly requested it. Other than that it was simply medication, medication, medication – with numerous side effects.
This is why it is important to me to shake things up with this book. First and foremost, I want to present the very positive results that I was able to achieve with natural medicine and complementary medicine. It is also equally important to me to make you aware of topics such as environmental toxins, pharmaceutical toxins, heavy metal toxification, overacidity and much more.

Why is the number of cases of Parkinson's disease increasing so rapidly in the Western world? Can we find any explanations in our lifestyle? Fifty years ago, Parkinson's disease was more or less unheard of in Africa and Asia. For a long time, even countries such as Denmark and Sweden did not experience the disease on the same scale as Germany and the USA. In Germany, the number of cases of Parkinson's disease is currently increasing by around 17,000 cases per year. In total the number of known and estimated undiagnosed cases in Germany is believed to be around 300,000. At the same time, the age of suffers is constantly decreasing. The youngest known sufferers are just 12 and 13 years old. Is this due to toxins in our environment, food and medication?

According to today's knowledge of the disease as described in conventional medicine, Parkinson's disease is a degenerative neurological disease. No truly curative treatments for Parkinson's have been made public at this point in time.
Why not? Because a truly curative treatment has not been scientifically proven?

My dear practitioners of conventional medicine, patients do not care whether a cure has been scientifically proven or not. They simply want to be healthy again.
I was given some pills out of the doctor's cabinet (without an information leaflet) and told, 'They're so new that even your pharmacist won't have heard of them.' Today I know that the effectiveness of these tablets was not scientifically proven and tested either, but instead, without realising, I had taken part in some of the pharmaceutical industry's studies.
This is why I appeal to all sufferers and their families: fight back! Do not let yourselves be patronised! Learn to make distinctions! It is vital for us all and for you especially.

# Part I

# Painful experiences
# Amazing findings
# Healing effects

## My life so far

### 1945

I was born prematurely at seven months under the horrors of the French-Moroccan occupation in a small village in Allgäu, Germany. My mother had been evacuated there from the heavily bombed Ruhr area. My father was in a Russian prisoner of war camp.
My premature birth was triggered by my mother being persecuted and raped by Moroccan soldiers.
At birth I weighed 1840 g. I was not expected to survive. An emergency baptism was performed and I was laid aside.
But, at my mother's insistence, I was brought to her; she was told that I did not have long to live anyway.
Obviously my will to live was already very strong! Because things turned out differently.

### 1947

We moved to the Ruhr area.
Nutrition was bad in general, and better described as makeshift.
There was a lack of everything.
Diseases.
The next kindergarten was only 100 metres from where I lived. I did not even need to cross the street. Yet after a few weeks I absolutely did not want to go any more.
My mother was worried and tried to find out why this was the case. It turned out that in this kindergarten, which was run by nuns, I was simply locked away sometimes – probably for being disobedient – in a pitch-black cellar which had the light-blocking doors that were still common at the time and were also airtight.

I can still hear the sound of the two heavy locks turning.

## 1952

Early diseases (rheumatism) due to lacking and insufficient nutrition, environmental toxins, lead pipes in the water supply, extreme pollution, etc. I was in hospital for months at a time due to rheumatic problems. I spent years on medication during my childhood and my time at school.

At that time, as is the case today, the side effects of medication were not considered. Advice from doctors was trusted completely. Despite this, I had loving parents who remained together and I felt comfortable and accepted.

I was always a quiet child, often withdrawn and absorbed in my own imagination. A teacher once said to my parents, 'Oh, I see your son sitting there and how he's in a world of his own. I just leave him be. I think he still knows what I've said.' Those were the people educating children back then!

Nowadays we know that children who are as quiet as I was could be suffering from ADD (attention deficit disorder). Back then this term had not been invented yet. Today children who disrupt lessons due to overly cheeky, hyperactive behaviour stand out. This is called ADHD (attention deficit hyperactivity disorder). However, today we also know that ADD or ADHD can be precursors to Parkinson's disease.


## 1953

The first signs of severe overacidity were ignored by doctors. Only a conscientious dentist explained to my mother where the black coating on my front teeth came from – from acids in the saliva.

This symptom still occurs in many children with ADHD today. Later in life this coating is attributed to natural causes such as tea, red wine or tobacco. It is no longer common to hear of 'overacidity' in conventional medicine.

## 1961

A severe bout of rheumatism meant four months in hospital with a course of injections and strong medication. Afterwards I was prescribed a two-year course of Resochin tablets as prophylaxis. I was also proscribed other medications with very strong side effects.

## 1964–1968

I completed my studies, received my degree and got married. I became self-employed straight away, setting up an office with my wife.

## 1971–2003

I held teaching positions as a lecturer at a university of applied sciences.

## 1972–2004

My wife and I had our own company and developed patents.
From the 1980s onwards, I was constantly having treatment for rheumatism and taking medication.

## 1973 and 1975

My two wonderful, strong-minded sons were born.

# I should have noticed

## 1995

I had strong, unexplained pain in both legs, back problems, outbreaks of sweat and dizziness. I experienced excessive, compulsive yawning whenever I went outside, for example during a walk in the woods. I asked a lot of doctors about it but they had no answers. These yawning attacks continued until 2008. I had headaches, dizziness and a constant feeling that everything was swaying, problems in the cervical spine, pelvic obliquity, a slipped disk and other problems.
… and always this pain.

## 1998

Due to a three-week-long viral infection I was temporarily unable to eat. I got through this period on baby food. This unexplained infection came back after almost exactly three months, then again after six months, and again the following year, but only for a few days.

## 1999

I had a slipped disk in the lumbar spine. Over the following years I had repeated medical spa therapy and took medication with side effects – i.e. toxins.
At one of the spa therapy centres there was no physiotherapist due to changes in staff. The doctor asked if I would also consider being treated by a Feldenkrais specialist. This was a fantastic 'coincidence'. It enabled me to learn a great deal about this unique kind of movement therapy. The young Feldenkreis teacher developed a special detoxification programme for me that I could do at home (see part III, Work sheets). I was also introduced to singing bowl therapy

for the first time.
At the end of my stay she also gave me the address of another
Feldenkreis teacher in my home town. This enabled me to carry out
the exercises once a week for many years under the supervision of a
very attentive, professional and helpful teacher, until I had to move to
a different town in 2005. This was a real shame, as I think further
treatment would have been highly beneficial.


## 2000

I suffered from dizziness, circulation problems, headaches and
increased hoarseness during presentations and lectures. The first signs
of memory loss appeared and I had problems concentrating.
I was no longer fit for daily life.
Medication, medication, medication!
I was often unable to remember the names of friends and
acquaintances when they were standing in front of me.
Now I know that the so-called transient ischemic attacks (small
strokes) that I had at night are malfunctions in the brain which are
signs of dementia.
What a shame that none of the doctors could explain this or treat me
for it directly.
Such information was recorded meticulously in my medical notes, but
nothing was done about it.
This constant tiredness and listlessness, this feeling of being out of
step, was very depressing.
The sensation of hearing myself speak as though it was someone
else who was speaking was highly unsettling.
At that time, after meetings and presentations I would say to my wife,
'During these discussions I feel like a politician who wants to answer a
question but usually never gets to the point and tells a different story
instead.' In politicians this is sometimes called diplomacy. In me it was
disease.

This time was a great burden for me. Sometimes I could not even remember the names of people I had known and worked with for years. I could not remember them at all. I now know that this was a manifestation of a severe liver disease. In alternative medicine this is considered a trigger or a cause of Parkinson's disease.

## 2003 – Unable to work

From 2003 onwards, I was unable to work and had symptoms that indicated Parkinson's disease which were first noticed by an orthopaedist. General practitioners and neurologists did not want to recognise the real problem, Parkinson's disease. A doctor of alternative medicine began a course of deacidification, heavy metal detoxification and oxygen therapy on me.
My GP dismissed these treatments as 'esoteric rubbish', a fatal error as I discovered later. I would have done better not to listen to him.
In July, I had a serious car accident due to lacking brain function. It became harder and harder to walk. As a consequence I had falls, I had ringing in my ears and I could not follow conversations. Reading required a lot of effort, as after a few lines I no longer understood what I had read.
I would have liked to have had Aslan therapy, a holistic therapy aimed at prevention and regeneration. My GP strongly advised me not to have it.

# 2004 – No research into the cause

## Rehabilitation

This was followed by a stay in a rehabilitation clinic.
By then it was already obvious that I had the typical gait of
someone with Parkinson's disease, but not for the doctor in charge.
I was prescribed more medication – along with all the side effects.

For all of the doctors who treated me then and over the coming years,
my complaints around my left temple and left cheek bone were rather
strange. I was told again and again that it was probably an
inflammation of the trigeminal nerve. In any case, according to 'expert'
opinion, neither of these complaints had anything to do with my
Parkinson's disease.
The same was said of the headaches at the top left of the back of my
head and the bottom left of the edge of my skull. Regarding the back of
my head, they simply said, '... you probably bumped your head there
once.'
It was not until four years later, during which time I experienced
constant severe complaints, that this incorrect diagnosis was cleared
up by a Vietnamese healer (see part I, Meridian seminar).

At the rehabilitation clinic I discovered that I could no longer walk
straight. I always veered to the right, no matter how hard I tried to
walk in a straight line. In this context, I remembered that over the past
few years my wife had pointed out how I tended to go the right when I
was walking.
The doctor in charge of the rehabilitation clinic thought that this was
due to a purely psychological reason. In her experience, she assured
me multiple times, it had absolutely nothing to do with Parkinson's
disease.

This doctor was clearly overwhelmed by her position as head of the clinic. I would like to illustrate this with the following unforgettable example.

As I had once again had severe back pain during my time at the rehabilitation clinic, I asked her for acupuncture after reading about it in the clinic's brochure. I did not want to keep taking the pain killers with their strong side effects. I wanted to be free from the pain without any more poisoning. I trusted that I was finally about to begin a treatment that would actually help.
The orthopaedist who had been treating me for years needed around 12 acupuncture needles which were put into my back for what felt like one minute.
The doctor at this clinic, on the other hand, needed what felt like one minute per needle and some of them were used several times in a very painful manner.
In the shoulder area she placed the needle so ineptly that I screamed from the pain. She simply said that she had probably hit a trigger point.
I was supposed to sit on the side of the treatment bed with the needles in my back for 20 minutes. Whenever I had had this treatment before I had always lain on my stomach.
After five minutes I felt so sick that I was swaying. I was worried that I would lose consciousness. I was scared that I would then fall back onto the needles.
With my last bit of strength I saw an emergency button in the treatment room and almost fell against it rather than lose consciousness. My last thought was, 'You have to fall forwards.'
After a while the clinic staff came and took out the needles and laid me on the treatment bed. As I threatened to collapse, the head of the clinic, the person who had caused my misery, was called. Her only comment was, 'Well then, I can't give you any more acupuncture. You're clearly not suitable for this treatment.'

To this day I have not received an apology for her lack of compassion and her weak acupuncture skills. Nevertheless, this experience did not have a long-term effect on my belief in the possibility of using acupuncture without any side effects. Acupuncture sessions carried out with skill by professional doctors and therapists have strengthened this belief.


## Deutsche Klinik für Diagnostik (DKD) German Clinic for Diagnosis

On my own initiative and at the recommendation of my orthopaedist who really did everything she could to help me, I made an appointment with the Deutsche Klinik für Diagnostik (DKD – German Clinic for Diagnosis) in Wiesbaden. I underwent a full examination there in the summer of 2004. The results: I did indeed have Parkinson's disease.

I was given more medication, but different and new kinds. It is worth mentioning an event with the psychologist at the DKD who gave me a form explaining how I could create a better future for myself through certain behaviour.

What shocked me in particular about this form was that, I quote, 'a small bad deed every day' was expected of me, in order to bring me out of my psychological low. I did not know what was meant by this. I showed this form to my doctors later who also reacted by shaking their heads in disbelief. At that time I could do nothing with the advice from this psychologist because I could no longer make decisions. My fear and apathy increased every day.

I just wanted to be left in peace.

# 2005 – A marathon of reviews and endless new medications

## Psychotherapy

My statutory health insurance provider recommended that I also take out additional private health insurance. I was happy to do so. However, I insisted that the additional packages also cover homeopathic methods and similar.

After the private and statutory providers had spoken to one another, my application was judged pointless as I was already being treated with a whole range of psychotropic drugs and it was therefore not possible for me to take out private health insurance coverage.
As the period of time for which I had been judged unfit for work was at an end, I no longer received any sick pay.
I subsequently spent a period of time struggling to have a disability pension extended. I was left with costs for many, many reviews. Costs for lawyers. Costs for courts.
A total of 19 reviews and medical certificates that all confirmed that I was unable to work due to my Parkinson's disease were required. I needed a great deal of help during this time.
I was at my wit's end.

I began psychotherapy with an unusually open-minded professor. Finally there was someone who took my complaints and struggles seriously. To this day I am thankful for these discussions, which provided explanations and showed understanding.

I was told that I was entitled to physiotherapy. First I had to tell this to the neurologist and request the treatment. I was then 'graciously' given two sessions a week, although not until autumn.

I kept bumping my head on things – strange. Everyone said that they could not understand me as my pronunciation was becoming increasingly unclear.
I kept experiencing these lows.
I could only read the newspaper for ten minutes, and after just five minutes I no longer understood what I had read. I also had unbearable headaches that never fully went away; I had ringing in my ears and my hands shook.
Muscle cramps in my whole body meant that I could only walk a few steps. Really it was just a slow shuffle. We thought about getting a wheelchair and a stair lift.
I simply could not go on.
I, a person who had made my own decisions all my life, who had often worked 20-hour days, 7 days a week, was now a wreck.
I discovered that my eyes started burning more and more often and the tears were aggressive. I was at a loss. The doctors I asked, specialists from various fields, did not have an explanation either.
At night during the sleep brought on by medication my legs were active, kicking and shaking. My handwriting became worse and worse. I was reluctant to write anything when I was being watched. I could barely read what I had scribbled myself anymore.
My wife had to help me dress and undress. Shirt buttons, socks and shoes in particular proved to be unmanageable hurdles.

# 2006 – The absolute low point

## Reviews

My application for a disability pension had to be justified in court.
The court decided on a specialist clinic for a final review – after the 17
reviews that had already been presented. The head of this clinic and
his team of senior staff who carried out the PET scan with injections
of radioactive contrast materials answered my question as to the
development and cause of the disease almost identically:
'Well, you known Muhammad Ali, the boxer, he has Parkinson's too.
He probably got one too many knocks to the head.' I replied, 'And
what about the pope?' (John Paul II who was pope at the time and
suffering from Parkinson's disease). 'That's probably a genetic cause.'
As I had done some research myself I simply could not believe the
way that patients were being treated as though they were stupid.
Unfortunately, I was no longer able to express this as I was unable to
form a coherent sentence due to my agitation. My wife had to
support me.
Later I often heard a similar explanation: 'It has psychosomatic
causes.' These are the standard phrases when doctors cannot or do
not want to give an answer.
This is often followed by 'You have to live with it now'. How can
they treat people like this?
To say they take people for idiots is putting it politely.

All of this might give the impression that I do not appreciate the
doctors' efforts.
This is not the case, and thankfully I have seen many times that
there are some fantastic, selfless and helpful doctors and medical
experts – often people in the emergency department, surgeons,
orthopaedists and specialists in many other areas of medicine.
However, I have also often felt that for some doctors I was simply a

member of a health insurance plan or someone with bothersome
requests. I was kept quiet with some kind of medication for the next
14 days, along with severe side effects, without compassion. If it did
not work I would be prescribed a different medication with a different
active ingredient. Throughout this process I was never asked about
any liver or kidney problems or other diseases. They were probably
not interested.
The main thing was that plenty of medication was prescribed.
However, I have to say that the doctors often simply did not have
any knowledge of the side effects of the chemical medications.
As medical degrees in Germany do not focus enough on the causes
of a disease, I think that they are simply unable to develop any
knowledge of this. I have the impression that nowadays treating
symptoms comes down to, in a nutshell: ask your pharmaceutical
representative.


## Court procedures

I tried to calm myself down, which was very difficult considering the
court date which had been set.
There were now 18 reviews and medical certificates that confirmed that
I was unable to work due to my Parkinson's disease and ruled out the
possibility of an improvement. Review number 19 also confirmed this,
but included a note saying that a completely different psychotropic
drug might make me fit for work again in a few years. The last review
was carried out by the pension insurance provider.
The doctor responsible, the head of a psychiatric clinic, had never
examined me, never seen me and never spoken to me. He had
judged my long-term illness 'on the basis of the files', as it is put so
cruelly.
The court was made up of one judge and four assessors.
I was at my wit's end when the judge, probably irritated and
annoyed by my tremor, said, 'Don't make such a fuss, nowadays
they just put a chip in your head and then you'll be able to work

again.' I had a nervous breakdown. My lawyer and my wife had to take me out of the court room.

When you consider that this court hearing was also about back payments from the disability pension amounting to several tens of thousands of euros – from the time the disease was recognised, so from 2004 onwards – the judge's brisk manner becomes more understandable. The representative from the pension insurance provider was more than happy with the judge.

I was no longer in a position to follow the proceedings. My lawyer was only able to get a settlement. Statutory pension insurance providers and providers of disability pension insurance in Germany are obligated to pay a disability pension from the moment when someone covered by the insurance is classified as unfit to work. In my case, this would have been after the examination by the DKD in 2004.

When is someone unfit to work in Germany? When a court has confirmed it. This can take years, as in my case, and can be delayed again and again by the pension insurance provider, until the person becomes so poor that they are willing to accept the solution presented to them.

Until then, you have no social security, i.e. no money, but are still obliged to make full payments to your health insurance and pension insurance providers – something I consider a huge scam.

Back at the beginning of 2005, the pension insurance provider had indicated to my lawyer that they would recognise my Parkinson's disease on the basis of the available reviews, if I was prepared to receive my old-age pension early, rather than a disability pension. For me this would have meant a life-long reduction of around 19 percent. As I did not agree to this since the overall loss, even if I reached the average age of life expectancy, would be too high, the pension insurance provider wanted to practically bleed me dry. On the basis of the files, the nineteenth reviewer from the pension insurance provider judged my Parkinson's disease as non-existent. However, on the basis of the same files, which had been going back and forth for years, he was of the opinion that I probably did have

Parkinson's disease but could be treated with a long-term stay in a psychiatric clinic.

So the pension insurance provider and the judge agreed that my entitlement would be recognised from 2004 onwards if I let myself be locked away in a psychiatric clinic.

I suspect that this was simply a way of scaring me. However, as I found this unacceptable, my lawyer was forced to agree to a settlement. My inability to work was recognised but not retrospectively. This saved the pension insurance provider a lot of money. I, however, was now in a very weak financial position and had to pay half of the court fees with the settlement money.

If I had not experienced it myself, I would not have believed the ignorance, incompetence and inhumanity with which I was treated by the court.

I accepted the settlement out of necessity.

From then on I understood: it was about my future, the future of myself and my wife; it was about activating the will to recover, to learn, to seek and find advice and information.

My findings are that diseases are not from God, as many religious communities are still taught from the pulpit. No, diseases are caused by people and their lifestyles – to some extent even before birth. I was afraid because the end, the true end, of Parkinson's disease is not being in a wheelchair, no, it is death through suffocation when the muscles can no longer carry out the brain's commands. This should motivate all sufferers to become healthy again or at least to lead a natural life which is worth living for longer.

## Prayer

In my distress and despair I found a quiet environment and prayed
what came into my head:

*God, our father, make me healthy again.*
*I know that would be a miracle now. But that is not what I mean.*
*Show me a path I can take.*
*Guide me to see things,*
*to get information,*
*so I can help myself through your goodness.*
*Give me knowledge, understanding and the will to help all people,*
*animals and plants.*
*Openness and tolerance,*
*love and compassion should fill me.*

And it was so!
Over the following years I experienced truly miraculous things which
I have written down here.
The book *Heilen verboten – Töten erlaubt* (healing forbidden – death
allowed) by Kurt G. Blüchel made clear to me for the first time the
relationship between practitioners of conventional medicine and
courts in Germany. Now I understood what the term 'sozial
verträgliches Frühableben'[1] (socially viable early death) used by the
former president of the German Medical Association meant in practice
for the individual.
This made me even more determined to seek solutions. After all,
we are not alone.
And there are no coincidences. We are guided. This is why the
following also apply here:

*FAITH, HOPE, LOVE.*

Think positively and do not forget to give thanks.
My new life had consequences. Tobacco and alcohol were banned.
As a layman when it came to medicine, I had to reorganise the world
for myself. But how can you do this when you no longer understand
anything and tiredness and pain define the day? Based on intuition I
began with the information included with my medication which,
trusting my doctors, I had not read until then. I was amazed at all the
things listed under the heading 'side effects'.


## Medication and side effects

*All of the following terms are taken from the information sheets included with the medications (originally in German).*

### Side effects of Mareen

Frequent: dry mouth, dry nose, tiredness, drowsiness, sweating, dizziness, drop in blood pressure, circulation problems, shaking, vision impairment, constipation, weight loss, increase in liver enzyme levels. Occasionally may cause problems urinating, restlessness, allergic skin reactions, sexual dysfunctions, confusion.
In rare cases may cause collapse, urinary retention, breast secretion, stimulation problems in the heart, accumulation of liquid in tissues, ringing in the ears, excessive dreaming, disruptions in hormone secretion in the pituitary gland, hair loss, changes in the blood glucose level, drug-induced hepatitis.
In isolated cases may cause seizures starting in the brain, increased pressure in the eye, complete enteroparesis and nerve dysfunction. Changes in blood count, sleep problems, problems swallowing, salivation, hand tremors, movement problems, fever, chills; inflammation in the nose, pharynx, mouth, genital and anal areas with itching may be a sign of a strong decrease in the number of white blood cells.

*Please note:* In patients with an organic brain syndrome the possibility that Mareen may be a trigger of confusion is to be questioned.


**Side effects of Stalevo**

Gastrointestinal bleeding, involuntary movement, nausea, irregular heartbeat and arrhythmia, dizziness, fainting, drowsiness, low blood pressure, sleepiness, sudden worsening of Parkinson's symptoms, loss of appetite, vomiting, development of a duodenal ulcer, stomach pains, dry mouth, constipation, diarrhoea, high blood pressure, inflammation of leg veins, insomnia, hallucinations, confusion, unpleasant dreams, tiredness, muscle cramps, excessive sweating, changes to blood cells and their components, fainting, infections, bleeding, shortness of breath, stomach pains, tingling and numbness, seizures.
Rare or very rare side effects: arousal, itching and rash, weight loss or weight gain, impaired vision, sexual dysfunction, among others.
I also read that particular care should be taken when taking the medication

If you have ever had a heart attack, asthma, vascular disease or lung
   disease
If you have or have had liver problems
If you have ever had a kidney disease
If you have ever had an adrenal gland tumour
If you have ever felt depressed or had suicidal thoughts
If you have ever had open-angle or narrow-angle glaucoma
If you have ever had a mental illness
If you are taking medication to lower blood pressure
If you experience involuntary movements during treatment
If you discover you experience severe muscle stiffness, strong
   twitching, shaking, arousal, confusion, fever or fluctuations in blood
   pressure

Mental health: mental anguish, increased appetite, occasional confusion, disorientation, hallucinations, anxiety, hypomania, personality disorders, aggression, memory and concentration problems, worsening depression and nightmares, activation of psychotic symptoms, among others.
Central nervous system: hand tremors, dizziness, headaches, muscle cramps, speech disorders, neuralgia and others.
Autonomic nervous system: dry mouth, sweating, blurred vision, urinary retention, among others.
Cardiovascular system: low blood pressure, high pulse, ECG changes, cardiac irregularity, among others.
Gastrointestinal tract: constipation, nausea, vomiting, diarrhoea, impaired sense of taste, thirst, rare ileus, among others.
Liver and bile duct: increased amount of liver enzymes, rare liver disorders, jaundice in rare cases, among others.
Skin and skin appendages: itching, photosensitivity, oedema and hair loss in rare cases.
Hormone system: sexual dysfunction, breast secretion in women, enlargement of mammary glands in men, menstrual disorders, among others.
Allergic reactions: pneumonia due to allergic reactions in rare cases, among others.
Blood formation: decrease in number of red blood cells, among others.
Sensory organs: occasional impaired sense of taste and ringing in the ears.
Other side effects: In the case of clomipramine infusions, isolated skin reactions may occur at the puncture sites. If the medication is discontinued without reducing it gradually, this may result in nausea, vomiting, diarrhoea, stomach pains, insomnia, headaches, anxiety and other side effects.

Notes for particular patient groups: Tricyclic antidepressants can reduce the seizure threshold meaning that seizures may occur in patients at increased risk of seizures due to epilepsy, brain damage, alcoholism, alcohol withdrawal, or concurrent use of antipsychotics.
… and so it went on.


**Side effects of Zolpinox**

Zolpinox has the same or similar side effect as the other medications listed, perhaps with a small difference – here there are many indications of memory problems, memory loss, depression, changes in behaviour, and physical and psychological dependence at various dosages.

This list could be extended almost endlessly and, in my opinion, shows only one thing: the flaws in the supposed blessing that is medication, not only with regard to the side effects in the affected organs but above all with regard to previous illnesses. The doctors who treated me never asked me about these, yet it is clear from these lists that these interactions can be incredibly important.
Why did the doctors not ask?

Other medications I took included:


Levodopa-neuraxpharm 100/25
Comtess 200 mg
Lorazepam dura 1 mg
Zopiclone-neuraxpharm 3.75
Doxepin-neuraxpharm 50
Fluoxetine beta 40
Fluoxetine-neuraxpharm 20T
Fluneurin 40 mg
and many more

Unfortunately I did not understand everything it said on these information sheets, but what I did understand shocked and disturbed me deeply.

What does the word 'medication' actually mean? The German word for medication, *Medikament*, has the following roots:

medica = to heal
ment    = mind
How far we have gone away from this! Who led us down this wrong path? In principle, it is this simple, as the mind heals us, the power of our thoughts, *without* chemicals, without side effects that cause sickness. But I did not understand this until years later.


## Psyche

There are certain kinds of nights that one does not want to experience. I remember a particular dream and experience. I am lying on a hospital bed and see only the tiles on the wall or floor. I am ice cold. I cannot move. It is as if I am frozen. I cannot call for help. I cannot do anything. I am petrified and I think 'NO! Not now!' Then, very slowly, my body warms up from my head down to my feet as if it is being passed through a scanner. It feels like this process takes over 10 minutes.

## Breuss treatment[2]

I now realised that I had to find a medication for myself. A friend, over 80 years old, who we had not seen in a very long time came to visit and seemed active and fresh, as if he were years younger. He told us about the Breuss treatment that he had done.
Rudolf Breuss was an Austrian practitioner of alternative medicine. Back in the 1950s, on the basis of natural observations and tests which he performed on himself, he was able to help and heal many people, in particular those with cancer but also people with many other diseases.
As my parents had died very young of cancer, my thoughts turned to this as well as my illnesses.
I sought out detailed information about Rudolf Breuss and his treatment, went to Nüziders in Austria and bought his book along with the vegetable juices and herbal teas that he had developed. My wife wanted to do the treatment with me, as it never hurts.
Mastering this extreme way of living together was a great support for me.
We carried out the treatment ourselves without supervision from a doctor. I had mentioned the subject to one of my doctors once. But he dismissed it. To not eat anything for 42 days – that seemed impossible to him.
Over the next 42 days there was nothing to eat. It sounds a lot worse than it actually was.
During the first three to four days it actually felt as if we were on a small diet. However, over the following days we began to feel better and better. During this time I lost a total of 25 kilogrammes. As I had become severely overweight due to the medication this was a positive result, but the most important part was the knowledge that I had purged all of the things that cause illness from my body.

The principle behind the Breuss treatment is to ensure that all substances in the body that cause illness, including those that cause cancer or cancer cells themselves, do not receive any more

nutrition. According to Rudolf Breuss, they can only survive on solid food.
During these weeks we drank the special teas that are part of the treatment at the required intervals. To prevent starvation, we drank the vegetable juice developed by Breuss and made by the Swiss company Biotta. As of 2008, they are now available in health food shops in Germany. Unfortunately the accompanying book is not. However, the new edition can be ordered from book shops.

We still do this treatment every year, often shortened to 8 to 10 days but sometimes for 3 weeks.

After the treatment I felt cleansed; I had the impression that my brain was more active, that I could somehow think more clearly. However, my problems when walking and my hand tremors had not changed. Something which I found particularly concerning was my problems swallowing, which usually also occurred at night.
My automatic swallowing reflex no longer worked, meaning that I was in danger of suffocating if saliva flowed into my airways, particularly at night.
Walking became more difficult and I became increasingly slower. The messages from my brain simply were not arriving in my legs.
However, thanks to the Breuss treatment, it soon became clear to me that nature offered ways and opportunities for me to regain my health. It was clear that my organs had been cleansed of toxic substances by the treatment. I trusted my instinct. I would receive information soon.


## Ayurveda

I found out about an Ayurveda practice located about 100 kilometres from my home through a newspaper article. They were having an open day. The new health centre, doctors, staff and treatments were being presented. We wanted to see it for ourselves. My wife and I

were very impressed, particularly as the very nice young Ayurvedic
practitioner from Kerala in India offered me an appointment for a
consultation the following week, which we gladly accepted.
What is Ayurveda?
The word Ayurveda means 'science from life'.
This medicine has been used for over 5000 years in India, making
use of over 3000 different herbs and mixtures. The standard length
of the training to become an Ayurvedic practitioner is five and a half
years. Ayurveda sees the person as a whole, as a unit made up of the
body and the soul. It considers the interactions between different
organ systems in the body.
In Ayurveda a person is seen as an open system which is constantly
interacting with its environment. The human body is in constant
flow; the interplay of material and energy constantly moves it from a
state of balance to unbalance and vice versa.
According to Ayurveda, full health can only be achieved through balance.
Regrettably, in Germany Ayurvedic practice has been largely relegated to
spa treatments. It is truly unfortunate that the incredible knowledge of all
these things is simply used for massages. Still, that did not bother me. I had
already learnt a reasonable amount about the possibilities and the
sometimes very drastic detoxification therapies and rough treatments. I was
willing to do anything if it would work.

Over the following week the consultation appointment drew ever closer. We
were surprised how pleasant and comfortable it all was. In addition to the
Ayurvedic practitioner there was a German alternative practitioner present
who had also studied and practiced Ayurvedic medicine in Kerala, India.
The initial consultation was about which treatments were
recommended and what could be achieved, so that an individual
treatment plan could then be made.
After we had discussed my medical history the practitioner began
with a pulse diagnosis in order to determine my energy flows and
constitution, i.e. my general condition and mental state.
The discussion and careful examination took almost 3 hours and

the conclusion was that it was possible to help me. In order to do so, I required a 30-day stay at the health centre with daily treatments.

The treatment could begin on the next new moon.

The practitioner asked for my permission to document my illness in writing and on video so that the various stages during the 30-day stay and the following 3 to 4 months could be presented to other patients with the same or similar illnesses.

I was hopeful. I was happy. Finally there was someone who could help me and actually wanted to do so, and they were going to do it using natural therapies as I had wanted.

For example, Ayurveda uses murdi thaila, a powerful herbal oil which is applied to the crown chakra, or a shirovasti, a head enema, is used to regenerate the nervous system and treat many other diseases. (For the head enema, a kind of open cap made of palm leaves, leather or a similar material is placed on the head and filled with special herbal oils. The oils penetrate the skin and their effects expand through the head.)

During a discussion with another Ayurvedic practitioner, kapikacchu (Sanskrit), a medicine made from Mucuna pruriens, was also mentioned. In Ayurvedic medicine it is considered a natural form of dopamine and is used to treat Parkinson's disease, restless leg syndrome and other diseases of the nervous system.

Over the next few days I was going to be told more about the exact nature of my treatment along with the suitable start date via e-mail.

I was very happy about this but I had not yet been given an estimation of the costs. I knew that this kind of treatment cost money, but how much? There were several phone calls. In the end it turned out that the treatment, including the cost of staying at the centre, would cost around 4 500 to 5 000 euros.

The staff at my health insurance provider did not consider this treatment to be scientifically proven, and therefore my health insurance could not pay for it or could only provide partial support.

I had more or less no money left. We had used up our savings over the last few years paying for living costs, court fees, various reviews from doctors and clinics, and lawyers' fees.

The court had denied me the pension I was owed by threatening psychiatric and pharmacological treatment. So there I was without any financial buffer to speak of.


## The end?

Was that it for my dream of a natural cure? After all, my health insurance provider only covered the pharmaceutical products which made me ill. In my case that meant swallowing 17 tablets a day with the side effects listed above, i.e. toxins that made me even more ill.


## Biliary colic

My gallbladder rebelled. Maybe it was because of this ridiculous medical policy?

While before the biliary colic had come at intervals of about three months, I now had it every week. Luckily I now knew from Breuss' book that a compress of warm horsetail (Equisetum) would relieve the pain within 15 minutes.

However, that was of course not a permanent solution.

I therefore decided out of necessity to go to a general practitioner. In the rather rural area where we live it was not yet common for GPs to own an ultrasound scanner, so the GP referred me to the nearest hospital.

The doctor there explained the ultrasound picture to me immediately. 'You have a gall stone there, about 17 millimetres in size. We should remove it over the next few days in a minor operation so that it doesn't cause you any more pain.' He turned the monitor towards me so that I could see it for myself.

I knew from my last check up at the DKD that I had had two 25-milimetre gall stones in 2004. The doctor who examined me then had also shown me the monitor. Due to the stones there was almost no space left in my gallbladder.

Of course I now told the doctor about this immediately.
The hospital doctor dismissed my statement completely. 'That's not possible. You must be mistaken. It's impossible for the stones to dissolve by themselves.' I knew that I had a real 'expert' here in front of me. I thanked him kindly for his efforts.
A few days after the discussion at the hospital appointment I brought the doctor my DKD documents, which explicitly mentioned the two large gall stones. The doctor could not or did not want to say anything in response to this and simply asked me whether she could copy the DKD report for her records.

Of course I wondered myself what had happened inside of me. I remembered that in the Breuss treatment that I had carried out myself several months before the key focus was the purification of the organs. Furthermore, I had been taking natural plant-based liver medication with natural vitamins and other compounds, including milk thistle, for several months. The stones clearly had dissolved and the larger pieces which were exiting my gallbladder had caused the colic in the bile duct. That was encouraging. So it really did work. There were ways in which I could help myself. I just had to find out what they were. I later discovered the methods of Dr Hulda Clark to be a very gentle alternative method of naturally removing gall stones without surgery.
It was not easy but I trusted that I was being led in the right direction. I just needed patience, it would work.

*Think positive     !*
*Set clear goals    !*
*Don`t complain   !*
*Don`t forget to be thankful !*

## Zapping

New research findings indicate that many diseases, even many kinds of cancer, often only have one major cause: parasites, bacteria, worms and similar.[3]

The Canadian medical practitioner Dr Hulda R. Clark has doctorates in cell biology (PhD) and naturopathy (ND). She has been working on cancer research for many years and has developed various devices, called zappers, which can eliminate causes of disease in the human body. Comprehensive information about the treatment also explains how and where, and in which organ these substances are present, be it the blood or brain. These are the causes of what we call lifestyle diseases.

According to Dr Clark, many cancers are caused by an intestinal flatworm in the liver along with the solution isopropyl alcohol and the clostridium bacteria. She believes that diabetes, for example, can be caused by the pancreatic fluke found in cattle present at the same time as methanol from solutions.

Dr Clark has found many common causes of various different diseases. It is important in every case, as it was in my own of course, to receive a detailed introduction to what should be changed in your life. You cannot get rid of the worms and other parasites but continue to consume cola, fast food, pork or other harmful substances in large quantities. Furthermore, the toxins in your house need to be identified and removed.

But let's start with the zappers. The first zapper that I got was the Dr Clark Full Gamma Generator. It is a direct current device which consists of a TENS (transcutaneous electrical nerve stimulation) stimulator made of two independent biofrequency generators. One biofrequency generates the sine wave and the other generates a square wave. Frequency, voltage and time settings can be set individually. The connection or contact is made using two cuffs on the wrists or ankles which are given the appropriate stimulation. It is simple and uncomplicated to use.

I began with the lowest setting and gradually increased the
frequencies over three weeks.
My digestion changed.
I felt my liver and large intestine 'working'. I then had a three-week
break, followed by three more weeks of treatment, and so on. This
purged my body of the undesirable 'inhabitants', the parasites,
worms, fungi, and similar mentioned above.
In this context I would like to recommend Dr Hulda Clark's book *The
Cure for All Cancers*. This work presents many causes of and
treatments for diseases, written in simple language so that the reader
is not left with questions. Partly in words, partly in diagrams, it
becomes clear what is toxic to our health in our everyday lives.[4]

For example:

| | |
|---|---|
| Acetone | contained in fizzy drinks |
| Benzole | in mineral water bottles and fruit juices |
| Carbon tetrachloride | in water bottles from supermarkets |
| Decane | in food and drink from health food shops |
| Hexane | in decaffeinated drinks |
| Hexanidione | in food with flavourings |
| Isophorone | in drinks with flavourings |

It also contains information on how to sanitise you house. To take one
example, in some buildings it is common for the garage to be integrated
into the ground floor. This is problematic for your health if your
bedroom lies above the radiation area of the car battery. According to
Dr .Clark, this will cause health problems.

Here are a few more tips:
Never drink hot drinks out of a Styrofoam cup, as the heat releases styrol.
Do not eat bread made for toast, as after toasting it you will be eating
benzpyrene and tungsten with it.
Do not use thermos flasks made of plastic, as the inside contains
lanthanides.

The toxins given in these examples are all present in small and minute quantities which are tolerated by law. Yet when we consider this more carefully, we should reject even the smallest quantities of toxins. In this great book we also find examples of what we can do better. For example, why we should not use deodorants and what alternatives there are. Why toothpaste which contains fluoride contains toxins but also what alternatives are available, and much more.

As a naturopathist, Dr Clark has researched what her ancestors in America, the Native Americans, used to regularly detoxify their bodies. The result of this research is – as all good things are – wonderfully simple. Three plants can free us from over 100 parasites. And this is without the interactions or harmful side effects we experience with many chemical products.

These three plant extracts are:
1. The green hull of the walnut from the American black walnut tree
2. Wormwood
3. Common cloves

According to this book, these three plant extracts can contribute to curing all kinds of cancer. Taken as prophylaxis, they purify the body completely so that its powers of self-healing are activated.[5]

**Back to the zapper:**
As part of her research on biofrequency, Dr Clark developed unique frequency treatments for specific diseases. There are over 70 types of what are known as programme drivers available – from acne to dementia, fibromyalgia, HIV, multiple sclerosis, Parkinson's disease, and tinnitus to viruses, dental diseases, and cysts.
Naturally, as part of my several weeks of therapy with the zapper, I also worked with the programme driver for Parkinson's disease. For me it was a problem that after just a few minutes I had very strong

headaches in the left side of my brain. I then did not use the driver
until several days later, and I used it more carefully and for a
shorter period of time. It was bearable but when I turned it up a
little the headaches signalled that it was better to take a break
again.
After several months of using it without the special Parkinson's driver I
began to feel itching on my wrists, meaning I could no longer put the
cuffs on for the therapy. I then put them on my ankles. This worked
just as well.
It was a shame that there was no distribution system in Germany at
the time which could provide information and assistance. To my
knowledge these issues in the initial stages of development have now
been dealt with.


## Water

I was experiencing circulation and heart problems, dizziness, anxiety
and cramps more and more frequently in addition to the common
symptoms.
I realised that I needed to reorganise my environment. I had to use
my new knowledge to steer my life towards a new path, one that was
beneficial to my health.
The human body is made up of at least 70 percent water. I learnt from
specialist literature that we should drink 40 millilitres of water per
kilogramme of weight per day. That means that, at 90 kilogrammes, I
needed to drink about 3.6 litres of liquid a day, such as water, herbal
tea and watered-down fruit juice.
Water is incredibly important for life and survival. We can survive for a long
time without food, but not even 5 days without water.
Water is soaked up by different parts of the body, such as the blood
and organs, and then expelled from the body along with toxins in the
urine. The intervertebral discs, the blood, the liver, the gallbladder,
the kidneys – all 80 billion cells of our bodies.

I already only drank still water such as Evian in order to avoid the acid of added carbon dioxide. However, I still needed a good alternative for washing, showering and boiling water for tea.

One of the first steps I took was to make my drinking water, i.e. tap water, drinkable and a better source of nutrition with a spring water generator. With new re-source technology, it is possible to give tap water the properties of spring water so that the water has a vitalising and purifying effect on our bodies. Isn't that a genius invention?

In recent years, it has been discovered that water has a kind of memory. The water molecules remember which electromagnetic waves and chemical substances they have come into contact with. This intelligent property of water has an influence on the water's structure, among other things. In nature, water molecules almost never occur alone. They form groups of molecules, known as clusters, in which many different $H_2O$ molecules join together in a wide variety of forms. By forming unique clusters of information and different energies, water can store almost unlimited data.

In this context I would like to make reference to the work of the Japanese researcher Masaru Emoto[6] whose books contain wonderful illustrations and information about the structures of tap water and spring water, lake water and other types of water. Considering these factors, it quickly becomes clear that the information stored in tap water often contains disharmonic information.

If allowing pure spring water to flow through 80 to 100 metres of constricting piping is enough to change it, it is logical that our drinking water network causes more and more changes to the water's molecular structure.

We know today, for example, that water from a spring on the surface is many times more valuable (almost a kind of healing water) than spring water which is pumped to the surface through pipes from hundreds of metres below and then sold as spring water, table water or mineral water. For this reason, one has to return tap water to its state as spring water, to reactivate its consciousness. Then the self-healing powers of nature will do the rest. In order to achieve this, inside the device there is a geometric structure, which is based on complex mathematical algorithms and principles from quantum physics.

To avoid creating false hope, I have to say that the device cannot remove toxins from tap water such as, for example, synthetically produced flurosurfactants which are sometimes found in drinking water in many regions.

However, it is helpful to know that the generator can have a positive effect on the large quantities of chlorine and fluorine added by water companies, the enormous pressure of the kilometres of piping and the ever increasing pollution due to electro smog. All of the toxic information is neutralised. The tap water re-energises itself in an entirely natural way. The lime scale stays soft and can be removed more easily. It is possible to use smaller amounts of washing powder and hygiene products. Tap water regains some of its purifying, cell-activating effects. For me, this is great for cooking and washing. However, I would not like to drink this tap water permanently. The pH value, which is much too low, and the pollution with additives change the rhythms in the water so much that I now only drink specific bottled water. Some brands of high-quality water include 7 Quellen from St. Leonhardsquelle, Evian or Volvic. Water with added healing minerals and/or $H_2O_2$ is also good.

# 2007 – I can begin to heal *without* chemicals

Illness is a lack of energy
What can a person do to calm themselves, to treat themselves, to make themselves strong again?
I started painting with oil paints again using a trowel technique. I had done this in the summer holidays of 2002. Don't get down, don't give up.
I thought of a quote by Albert Einstein:

*The purest form of insanity is
to leave everything the same
and at the same time to hope
that things will change.*

So you need to move, but in the right direction!
You cannot keep repeating what is convenient and familiar. There is so much to discover and experience. It is important to think positive. Everything that I am is only a result of that which I have constructed. It always comes back to me; the positive thoughts and those that make me ill.
What causes disease?
The body becomes ill due to hunger or viruses. A carefully considered diet and good water bring balance.
The soul becomes ill due to dreams. Reflection and psychotherapy can help here.
Loss of energy occurs due to blockages which must be removed. If our energy field is weakened, it is likely that we will become ill.
The invisible layer of energy that surrounds us is known as the aura. People who can perceive this are able to read it like an open book.
So many insights, but where should I begin?

## E numbers

Now when I go shopping I always take a small book with me which lists all of the currently known E numbers. E numbers on packaging indicate the natural and chemical additives in food. Two thirds of the products that I pick up I end up putting back on the shelf.
It is truly extreme how many chemicals we unconsciously expect our bodies to take. The average amount per person in Germany is around three kilogrammes per year of these toxins – whether they are a baby or a senior citizen. For this reason, I am even stronger in my conviction to only buy things which I can eat and drink with pleasure. E 104 chemical colourings are thought to contribute to ADHD, for example. E 128 is categorised as carcinogenic. The E numbers 249 to 251 are known to cause the formation of carcinogenic nitrosamines. With regard to cheese and other milk products, I look for unpasteurised products. While items that have been pasteurised or heat-treated may be tasty too, they unfortunately no longer contain the full power of all the vitamins and minerals.
The same applies to rice. Experts prefer brown or red whole-grain rice, from the Camargue in the south of France, for example, or brown rice from Japan – the full power of nature!

I also always take a small book about products and their acid-base balance with me. When shopping it is important to check whether products really are as basic as you think. It is often not the case. I still have a lot to learn. Nevertheless, this topic is so important that it is worth changing your perspective immediately and getting used to this form of nutrition.[7,8]

## Singing bowls

We visited Paris in January and one of the places we went to while we were there was the Louvre. Once again, by 'chance', alongside the Tibetan exhibition which was running we saw Tibetan singing bowls in the museum gift shop. I remembered the very beneficial treatment with singing bowls that I had received from a Feldenkrais practitioner. I decided to buy myself one of these singing bowls. But which one? The range on offer was not too large but it was still difficult for a layperson. I trusted my instinct and simply took the one that sounded the nicest to me and which had the most pleasant vibration. This singing bowl had a light tone. Strange, because I usually preferred the darker tones, but I stuck by my decision. Intuitively, I immediately used it where I had the most problems: my head, the control centre for all orders. It was not until a year later, at a workshop on how to carry out singing bowl therapy, that I learnt from the course leader that the singing bowls with the high notes are very helpful for all problems with the brain. He said that special vibrations that are even finer and more effective can be particularly helpful here.
Today I know that I am stimulating my lymphatic system to remove all the toxins from my body every day with these vibrations. I thank my intuition for making the right decision!


## Moving house

We had moved near Baden-Baden. The temperature in the warm countryside in this area was 8–10 °C higher than in the Ruhr area. That was very pleasant. Here we also had the opportunity to go to the wonderful thermal baths once or twice a week.
The nights were restless. I was plagued by dreams which were sometimes violent. My legs and arms were constantly moving. It was not just me who was bothered by this. My wife did not get any rest either. They were simple muscle reflexes that were partially controlled by the brain. Certain symptoms were caused by the nervous system.

Many years later in the magazine *Welt der Wunder* (September 2010 issue) I read about a study which proved that 80 to 100 percent of people with these kinds of dreams either suffer from an acute disease of the nervous system, such as Parkinson's disease, or certain kinds of dementia, or would do within a few years. Again and again, sufferers dream that they must fight off attackers. However, because the muscles are not relaxed as in a healthy person, the muscles react directly. This sleep disorder is called RBD, REM sleep behaviour disorder.

My condition then deteriorated suddenly, once again making me incredibly disheartened and demonstrated the problems of Parkinson's disease right before my eyes.

I could barely walk. It was as if I was frozen and I could not even turn over in bed. My muscles did not respond to my commands.

I started from the beginning again.

At this stage the neurologist told me that she could only prescribe me physiotherapy once a week now due to the healthcare reform.

Don't give up, practice slowly.

The knowledge I had gained during many years of Feldenkrais therapy was very beneficial here. However, the physiotherapy also helped my movement, which was still very limited. Everywhere I looked I saw and received tips and information.

I just needed to be more patient!


## Colloidal silver

I found out for the first time during certain discussions that Parkinson's disease can often be caused by problems in the intestine.

Colloidal silver is effective against germs, bacteria and fungi. It has been used as a natural remedy for humans, animals and plants for over 5 000 years. In ancient times, silver was used to speed up the healing of wounds, to fight infection and in particular to preserve drinking water. Colloidal silver is a natural antibiotic that has been increasingly pushed out of the market since chemical antibiotics have become available since the 1930s.

When penicillin was discovered the use of colloidal silver stopped almost completely. However, in the early 1990s, it became more and more widely known that certain strains of bacteria were building up a resistance to pharmacological antibiotics. In light of this, silver began to regain significance as an additional and alternative treatment.

Colloidal silver consists of minute silver particles dissolved in water. It may be used as an additive in food under the name E 174.

As I was searching for ways of detoxifying the intestine this was one of the first important discoveries that I made.

Its effects were noticeable but did not remain stable in the long-term in my case, causing me to continue my search. However, for simple stomach and intestinal diseases, if used correctly, its antibacterial effects can be very beneficial. Bone growth is also accelerated by silver.[9]

## St John's wort oil

I use St John's wort oil for spine massages, for daily massaging of the liver and spleen area, and for stomach lymph drainage. The type that clearly works best for me is Breuss St John's wort oil. As I need large quantities of it, this year I decided to make it myself.

St John's wort grows on the edges of woodland and farmland. Large numbers of these small yellow flowers can be found in June (24 June is St John's day) and, depending on the weather, through to July and the start of August. The flowers, which blossom at the end of June, are very suitable and should be picked when the sun is shining. St John's wort oil and other St John's wort products should not be used if you also plan to spend time sunbathing as it makes the skin more sensitive to the sun's rays and you can quickly become sunburnt.

Tip: Before sealing the bottles, you should pour a small amount of clear alcohol (at least 40 percent) carefully on top of the oil to make the seal airtight. The oil will keep for two to three years. If you decant it into smaller bottles in between, you should shake it well first so that the alcohol mixes with the oil. After you have decanted what you need for the next few weeks it should be 'resealed' with alcohol.


## Pendulum

*'I want to keep things as simple as possible, but no simpler.'*
(Albert Einstein)

During this phase, the pendulum motion caught my interest. Without making a big deal about it, a dear friend of mine would use a pendulum on objects that lay in front of him while we were eating or shopping. To start with I found this very odd. However, I was happy for him to explain it to me and learnt that he was using the pendulum to measure the energies, or rather the vibrations, of the objects around him.

These energies are measured in Bovis units. The physicist André Bovis (1871–1947) came from Nice. He developed a biometric scale that was later improved and calibrated by the electronic engineer Simonéton. The measurement results that can be compared with one another have since been called Bovis units (BU).
At the time I was learning and discovering how important it is to only consume food and drink with a high energy value and I wanted to know more. I knew that food and drink had to be valuable, but how did you determine what was valuable? According to our experience we know that information provided in advertising for food and drink is not to be trusted. This is designed to sell, but I want to eat foods which are rich in energy. The two are not compatible.

I read the book *Rute und Pendel* (rod and pendulum) by Gertrud I. Hürlimann with great interest and several things became clear to me. The use of pendulums or, more specifically, radiesthesia has been practiced for thousands of years, whether in Ancient Egypt or Ancient Greece (Oracle of Delphi). There are reports from the last few centuries of people who knew the art of the pendulum. Among them were Johann Wolfgang von Goethe, Albert Einstein and many others.[10]

As a principle, I will never use the pendulum for questions of fate. For me it is only about determining the scientific energy values of my food and my own wellbeing with the help of the pendulum. All materials are in vibration and therefore have measurable electromagnetic wavelengths. The intensity of their radiation can be determined with the Bovis biometer and measured in Bovis units. A neutral value is 6500 Bovis units, sometimes called bioenergy units (BU). When this value is divided by 10 you get the unit which is used in physics today for wavelength: the nanometre (nm). Therefore, the example given about is 650nm. However, when using a pendulum, the Bovis unit is usually used to ensure clear, uniform values for comparison.
Starting with the neutral value of 6500 BU given above, this is measured for natural fertile soil, for example. A healthy living space and edible food should have values that lie above this average. Everything below this value lacks quality. The energy balance of a healthy person has a value of between 7000 and 9000 BU. If a person becomes ill they have less energy. This is then very clear in the energy value measured.
The principle is similar for food. Lower values of below 6500 BU indicate how inferior these things are and how damaging they are for our strength. We would do better not to eat or drink these things. Items with higher values starting at around 7500 BU can truly be considered real food.

Below are some examples based on the knowledge I have gained from this. The results of the measurements are simply examples and you may wish to check them yourself.

| | |
|---|---|
| Industrial bread | approx. 4000 BU |
| Bread from a bakery | approx. 8000–10000 BU |
| Home-made bread for which you have also ground the grain yourself and used natural yeast or sourdough | approx. 12000–14000 BU |

| | |
|---|---|
| Honey from a discount supermarket | approx. 5000 BU |
| Honey from a beekeeper | approx. 10000 BU |
| Honey from a beekeeper with added pollen | approx. 14000 BU |
| Honey from mountainous regions, by the treeline, etc., Italy, Switzerland | approx. 27000 BU |

| | |
|---|---|
| Plain mineral water | approx. 3500 BU |
| Good still water such as Volvic or Evian | approx. 7500–9000 BU |
| St. Leonardsquelle, Lichtquelle | approx. 13500 BU |
| St. Leonardsquelle, Sonnenquelle | approx. 16500 BU |
| Spring water after 3 hours | approx. 1250 BU |
| Spring water with $H_2O_2$ | approx. 16500 BU |
| Tap water on average | approx. 5000–6000 BU |
| Tap water in a Swiss mountain village | approx. 8000 BU |
| Tap water in Lourdes (France) | approx. 11000 BU |
| Lourdes water | approx. 26000–30000 BU |

This list could be extended indefinitely. It shows how exciting the topic is.

Try testing some things for yourself, such as margarine, crisps, fast food, lemonade, chocolate bars, schnapps or cigarettes. You will see that it is worth looking for high-quality, energy-rich foods and drinks, and for organic fruit and vegetable juices. Only by doing so can you become healthy and stay healthy.

The slightly stunted apple or the small, unimpressive orange suddenly becomes the most appealing, not due to pity but because of the knowledge that you are eating something healthy with good energy.
Everything should be measured. Take a look at personal hygiene products, such as soaps, creams, perfumes and deodorants. All medications, flowers, healing stones, etc. can also be measured. Remember that our skin is our largest organ. Any bad or low-quality products that we put on our skin have a long-term negative effect on our entire bodies. This is why all new products should be tested with the pendulum in order to determine which is better.
However, questions do not always have to be about Bovis values. The pendulum can also be used for other questions. For example, you can use a percentage scale to determine by how much certain foods, supplements, medications, etc. can help. When a friend of mine asked me to determine the Bovis value of her arnica globules I made a surprising discovery. Arnica C 30 globules have a Bovis value of around 64 000 BU! Now I knew what an incredible potential for healing was in these homeopathic globules. It is also easy to answer basic questions that can be answered with yes or no. It is very simple. You just have to do it. I have learnt to make distinctions. It's fun too. Try it! You will see that success will prove you right.[11]

## Stevia

The sweet herb stevia is found across South America and China. Stevia contains almost no calories and has health-boosting properties. It is a very good alternative to harmful sweeteners and white sugar (granulated sugar).
The plant extracts used as a sweetener do not form harmful carbohydrates in the body and do not have an effect on blood sugar levels as granulated sugar does. Diabetics can therefore use it without any concerns. Finally there is an alternative to harmful chemical sweeteners.

I was recently given a stevia plant by a friend which now stands on my balcony. Now I can simply pick what I need each day. In addition, for the past few years I have only been using natural unrefined sugar. Yes, the kind which sticks together if you do not use it for a few days. I like this; it is like a kind of seal of quality. Finally a food that does not contain large amounts of aluminium or nanoparticles!

These findings are crucial, as people suffering from Parkinson's disease or dementia have heavy metals in the brain which cause blockages in the nerve cells so that commands like walking or picking up a cup cannot be carried out. Aluminium is classified as a heavy metal in medicine.

In Germany there are no legal regulations on certain additives in food such as aluminium, nanoparticles and citric acid from the black mould Aspergillus niger. Why not? I probably no longer need to mention the advantage of stevia in comparison with industrial sugar or chemical sweeteners, which contain substances such as aspartame. This is finally being brought to people's attention in the media by courageous journalists.

Please find out about this. It's for your health![12]


## Permanent ear acupuncture

I read about the methods of Dr Werth that were used to cure Parkinson's disease through permanent acupuncture in the ears in the magazine *Fliege* (issue 12/2007).[13] Dr Ulrich Werth spent time practicing medicine in Valencia, Spain. The success rate of his methods was apparently 80 percent.

I heard about a specialist acupuncture practice in Niedeggen from another Parkinson's sufferer. There Dr Thomas Schockert carries out ear acupuncture, as well as scalp acupuncture, using the methods of Toshikatsu Yamamoto, known as Yamamoto New Scalp Acupuncture (YNSA). I heard about these possibilities but did not try them myself.

## Human and Universal Energy®

Something had to change!

I felt as through, despite all my physical and psychological problems, I *wanted* to change something.

An old saying says 'If you want to change something, you have to start with yourself.'

A good friend of mine told me about Human and Universal Energy®. I trusted him and listen carefully to what he said to me. He spoke about people who explain and teach how you can support the healing processes with the inexhaustible energies of the universe and develop the ability to help other people to confront their everyday lives with greater physical and mental strength. You start with yourself and then move on to people in your family and later to anyone who wants help.

'These people help without any ifs or buts,' my friend explained. 'They are guided by their love and their compassion for their fellow human beings, animals and nature. Their energy transfers are always free. They do not make any distinctions between different cultures, skin colours, religions or nationalities. They help by transferring energy – just because, without getting anything in return. Anyone can ask.'

I was beyond curious and decided to take my first seminar.

On a rainy weekend in October I sat with the other participants in the seminar room and listened with fascination. During the breaks and at dinner I got to know the other participants better. I was very surprised at the range of professions that I met here. There were students, nurses, midwives, doctors, housewives, teachers, architects, healers, physiotherapists, foresters and animal breeders from Germany, Switzerland, the Czech Republic; the list goes on. I asked everyone why they were taking part in the seminar and how they had found out about it. I had a particularly intense discussion with one participant. This man openly told me his story. Five years ago he had suddenly developed a disease in both eyes. Over the following years he had lost 90 percent of his vision. He underwent various eye operations – with the result that he had regained some vision after the last operation and now had 20 percent. The doctors were very satisfied. However, he and his wife kept looking. They simply did not want to settle for this. They had been given the address of a woman in a neighbouring town who used a special technique to transfer universal energy, helping people a great deal. During our conversation he fought back tears, full of happiness and thankfulness. He said that thanks to her help his vision had increased to 80 percent. The doctors at the specialist clinic were baffled. He was happy. He wanted to take part in the seminar so that he too could help people in the future.

Years later I saw him again at an advanced seminar. This time he was accompanied by his eye doctor who also wanted to undergo this training for himself and for his patients.

I heard the stories of many people's fate during this time, but I have to say that this one had the most profound effect on me. The wonderful opportunities that this huge amount of energy makes available to us can only be met with great thanks, happiness and love.

It was a wonderful experience! But it changed us. We learnt how important it is to see people, animals and nature through different eyes. We learnt techniques to transfer this energy from the universe to people and animals, but also to nature, to trees and fields, for example. We learnt to help anyone who asked us to. We learnt to fill our lives in a different way, to get rid of stress and deal with everyday challenges in a more relaxed way. Love and compassion for others were at the heart of it.

Over the time we became noticeably more balanced, more willing to help, and happier. We set new priorities and gained a new perspective when interacting with other people. Things that were important before were given a new value, as we moved our attention away from selfish, insignificant and worthless actions.

The founder of this wisdom and practical knowledge was the
Vietnamese master Luong Minh Dang (1942–2007). The training
programme is called Human and Universal Energy®. Master Luong
Minh Dang's original programme is dedicated to a holistic approach to
the relationship between the body, mind and soul.
It was the sincere wish of the founder of this training programme that
by using the techniques and information we would be able to achieve a
state of wellbeing. The programme focuses on activating our chakras,
the body's energy centres. Activating our chakras allows us to use
universal energy effectively and transfer it to ourselves and other
people.
During the seminars participants are taught the skill of transferring
this universal energy with the hands during meditation. The
information and techniques taught here can be applied immediately in
your professional and private life. You can immediately begin to
support yourself, your family, your friends, colleagues and employees,
and your environment in a new way using energy.
I can personally say that this conscious way of living inspired me
greatly and has significantly improved my health for the long term.
I am always pleased when an opportunity arises to help other people.
Unfortunately, I have also experienced that not all of my family and
friends understand what happened here with me and later also with
my wife.
This method is not a medical treatment! When we look at the
media today, we can be confident that the future of people in this
century will make a giant leap towards activating the power of self-
healing through meditation.
I believe it is time that society changed its way of thinking.

## Atlas correction

At a seminar that is often attended by people from all over the world my attention was drawn to another therapy known as atlas correction. The atlas is the top most, i.e. the first, cervical vertebra of the spine which holds up the skull. The connection between the skull and the atlas is out of place in almost all people in our society due to various aspects of our lifestyle.
Due to this displacement the hole in the skull and the vertebral canal are made smaller so that nerve and lymphatic tracts, as well as various blood vessels in the spinal canal, are constantly under pressure. This can cause problems ranging from pelvic obliquity, hip problems, scoliosis, neck pain and general back pain to meniscus problems and other knee problems, but it can also cause mental health problems. Atlas correction stimulates and supports the body's self-healing and regeneration processes in the long term.
This correction is carried out using the method developed by René C. Schümperli in Thun in Switzerland. What is special about this therapy is that it only needs to be carried out once in a person's lifetime. It never has to be repeated – unlike many of the treatments that are often offered in Germany.

My wife and I were sceptical, but we had our atlas vertebrae aligned. The correction was painful for one or two minutes but after that it did not hurt.
Within a few weeks, the first effect was that our legs and pelvises were realigned. Up until then we had always had to shorten one of the legs after buying a new pair of trousers – this leg was now too short. Before then the heels of our shoes had always worn down unevenly; now the wear was only minimal and almost straight and in the centre.
I think this therapy also helped me to place my feet better and more evenly in the long term, as the characteristic gait for Parkinson's sufferers is to walk on the outer edges of the feet. Walking more evenly, however, gives more stability and decreases the risk of falls.

At our age – in light of the illnesses we had been carrying around for decades – the repositioning of our entire bodies took several years. However, the crucial point for us was that it got a little better every day, and continues to do so today.

In the follow-up discussion with the therapist where we discussed my Parkinson's disease, I was told about two books by Dr Peter Jentschura and Josef Lohkämper, *Zivilisatoselos* (free from lifestyle diseases) and *Gesundheit durch Entschlackung* (health through detoxification).[14]

The book *Zivilisatoselos* lists almost 60 diseases which, according to the authors, are largely lifestyle diseases and can be cured using natural methods. It seems unbelievable, but it is true.

I bought these books and studied them like bibles. The best thing I learnt was that Parkinson's is also one of these lifestyle diseases and therefore can also be treated with these simple but very effective methods of active deacidification and basic living; an important prerequisite for healing, regardless of the disease.

I admit that it can be tiresome, as my weekly alkaline baths still take a good hour and a half today. In the beginning, the alkaline enemas and rinsing the frontal sinus and the oral mucosa require a lot of time. But when all of this is to cure Parkinson's disease, it is an easy chore that I gladly undertake. After all I have one goal: I want a healthy and active life again.

I will be forever grateful to these authors for their revolutionary yet so simple methods of alleviating suffering and contributing to healing (see part II, chap. 1, Possible causes of Parkinson's disease; chap. 2, Possible therapies for Parkinson's disease).

## Magnetic field therapy

Magnetic field therapy is mainly used as method of treatment in orthopaedics and sports medicine, but it should also be used to treat other kinds of illnesses. It has an effect on the whole body. To my knowledge, stimulation of the nerve cells through magnet field therapy promotes faster nerve cell regeneration in all neurological diseases, such as Alzheimer's disease, multiple sclerosis, Parkinson's disease and depression.

The brain essentially functions like an electronic system; information is transported via electrical impulses between cells. These processes can be influenced by magnetic fields. Researchers hope to be able to help people with neurological diseases in this way. Their goal is to animate the healthy parts of the brain to take over the functions of the defective brain regions.
However, these effects can be felt across the whole body. For example, bladder function can return to normal if there are bladder problems. The healing process after surgery can also be accelerated with magnetic field therapy. The feeling of exhaustion that is common in Parkinson's disease is compensated for. Tremors in particular, but also muscle stiffness, improve to an extent. In terms of mental health, magnetic field therapy aims to make depression and anxiety bearable. I did not use this therapy myself because I had chosen other methods. However, I feel it is work mentioning as something which may hopefully be helpful to sufferers.[15, 16]


## Meridian seminar

I was visiting friends in Switzerland. We wanted to go to see a Vietnamese healer together who had a treatment centre near Lucerne. The weekend seminar taught about treating the meridian points with universal energy.
Mr Thai Ngoc-Buu is an extraordinary man with, I had heard, extraordinary success in healing. We were greeted by a warm,

caring man. Without having seen him before, you knew instantly that it was him.

Mr Thai used images to present the human body with the meridians which run through it and the associated acupressure points. Practical examples followed. There were around 80 to 90 participants at the seminar listening to his explanations. When he spoke you could have heard a pin drop; everyone was hanging on his every word. I found it highly interesting. As he spoke Swiss German it was not always easy for me to understand everything, but my friends helped if something was unclear.

Mr Thai explained to us the relationships between everyday things that make us ill and the result that our meridian points sometimes become very painful.

Meridian treatment has been around for thousands of years but is almost unheard of in the German-speaking world, especially in combination with universal energy. The aim of this seminar was to give us the ability to activate our powers of self-healing and those of other people through specific methods in the future.

Of course the question I was keen to ask was what the right meridian points are for Parkinson's disease.

Mr Thai had clearly already worked out why I was there. He smiled and asked me where I was currently feeling pain. I explained to him and the other participants that it was at the bottom left edge of my skull. I remembered that I had been suffering from this for years and had mentioned it to all of my doctors, who told me, 'You probably bumped your head there.'

Now Mr Thai's explanations opened my eyes. He explained to me that there is a small dimple on the bottom edge of the skull which can be felt on both the left and the right. Everyone touched the backs of their heads. Yes, we could all feel them. If, like I was, you were experiencing pain in this area, the pain would ease if you rubbed and pressed lightly in this area. The trembling in my hands would also decrease or even stop completely with a bit of practice!

A complementary method of manual therapy from Mr Thai is to simply

concentrate on this point during meditation. The back left edge of the head is connected to the right hand and the right leg, and vice versa; back right edge = left hand and left leg.
Good to know. I no longer had to endure doctors smiling at me and making me feel like I was crazy.

I immediately began to include these methods in my daily programme, with the result that after four weeks the pain was gone and after several months even the tremor was too. Of course the seminar went into much more detail. We learnt ways in which we could awaken the powers of self-healing in ourselves and our fellow human beings. According to Mr Thai, this is possible through the energies that the universe makes available to us and which simply need to be called upon. In my experience it is very simple. You just have to do it. It works, as I was able to experience myself, for everyone.
Mr Thai gave us all a little black stick. This was first to be used to stimulate the central point of our nervous system on our skulls. (This point lies exactly where the line between the two ears and the line between the nose and the spine cross; a small dimple on the skull can also be felt here.) We later practiced the procedure on other participants as well to be sure that we could find exactly where this point is. For most of us it was a wonderful, relieving sensation to feel this. Since then, my wife and I have done it every day.
It was a fantastic weekend. We learnt a lot. All of the participants were agreed on why this healing method has not become part of conventional medicine. Incidentally, there were also doctors, healers and other healing professionals there. In Switzerland people are usually very open to these experiences (see part II, Meridian therapy). During this year I learnt a lot about how I could train and refine my feeling of health. For example, I began to attend homeopathic seminars to educate myself. I continued to do so intensely over the following years, with workshops and training sessions on Schüßler salts, Bach flower remedies, energy transfers and vibration/energy medicine.

There is a lot to do.


## Schisandra berries

The schisandra berry is known from the oldest Chinese compendium of healing plants, *Pharmacopeia of the Heavenly Husbandman Shen Nung* (around 2600 BC.).[17] It is a small red berry which, similar to the cranberry, is like a grape but grows on vines. There must be something to the almost 5000-year-old reputation of its healing powers, I thought to myself.

In China great value has always been placed on these berries as a kind of prophylaxis but also for medical problems. The schisandra berry is called wu wei zi. This means 'the plant of five tastes'. This is because it tastes sour, the hull and flesh are sweet, but the pips are sharp and sometimes bitter, and all of the parts together leave a slightly salty aftertaste. The berries are rich in vitamin A, vitamin C, vitamin E, vitamin B1 (riboflavin), vitamin B3 (niacin), vitamin B6 (pyridoxine), as well as the minerals calcium and iron, and trace elements such as selenium, iodine, tin, cobalt, phosphorus, potassium and sodium.

The berries and their nutrients have a balancing effect on the body as a whole. This means that the berries improve physiological functions. For example, if blood pressure is low, it is increased. If blood pressure is high, it is decreased to a normal level. Over-sensitivity is balanced out. Brain activity is stimulated, counteracting forgetfulness. The liver, gallbladder, spleen, heart, lungs, large intestine, bladder, kidneys, eyes, ears, bones – in short the entire body is affected.

In the mid-twentieth century, researchers in the former USSR were tasked with studying these berries, which had been unknown in Europe until then. The research project was led by the doctor, researcher and pharmacologist Nikolai V. Lazarev and his colleague Israel I. Brekhman.

Over time the group of researchers in Russia grew to over 1200 scientists. There were over 3000 clinical trials with over 4000 different healing plants. The best results were achieved in experiments with the schisandra berry. Due to these outstanding results, the crème de la crème in the world of sport and culture (such as the Bolshoi Ballet), as well as world chess champions and the military, were given these berries. They were used anywhere where stamina, concentration, the utmost alertness and high productivity were required. According to my experience, for Parkinson's sufferers they offer a natural way of stabilising brain function and allowing the body and mind to cooperate harmoniously again. This is largely due to glutathione, the most important antioxidant in the brain.

The schisandra berry is able to raise glutathione levels in the brain, limiting production of free radicals and increasing antioxidant protection of the brain.

In Japan there is already a patent for the use of active agents in schisandra berries to treat Alzheimer's disease by reducing beta amyloid deposits.

The schisandrins contained in the berries also offer good protection for livers which have been damaged by certain medications. The berry is successful against all neurodegenerative diseases, such as multiple sclerosis, Alzheimer's disease and Parkinson's disease, as these diseases are associated with very low glutathione levels.

For Parkinson's sufferers, these factors mean that, due to the effect of glutathione, the messenger substance dopamine is able to stimulate the dopamine receptors, meaning that even reduced dopamine production can be used better. Certain glutathione therapies can show considerable decreases in symptoms such as tremor and rigor (the almost mechanical, cog-like arm motion). The schisandrins in schisandra berries can be a great help here.

Parkinson's disease is caused by cell death in the substantia nigra – an area in the centre of the brain in which the messenger substance dopamine is produced. The antioxidant effect of the glutathione contained in schisandra berries is able to considerably reduce the symptoms of Parkinson's disease.

Schisandra berries are available dried in Germany. You can buy them online or try asking at an Asian supermarket. Make sure to check their freshness. While the berries are always dried, they should be about the size of a juniper berry and still soft when squeezed. Berries that are only the size of a peppercorn are too old and too hard. Ground or grated schisandra berries should also be avoided, as they lose much of their effects due these processes.

The rarer schisandra berry variety known as wu wei zi is only found in one particular province in China and is unfortunately not available in Europe. However, if you have contacts in China you may be able to get them from there. I recommend them as their effects are even stronger – my pendulum confirms that they have a very high Bovis value. Alternatively, you could plant some yourself in your garden. The plants can survive through winter. Contact a garden centre or look for a specialist online.[17] I still use dried berries, usually the wu wei zi which are available for delivery to Germany, every now and again for a two to three month treatment.

# 2008 – Accepting and overcoming setbacks

The year did not start well.
During the first few days I once again had these dreams and
experiences of reality that I had had at the end of 2006. I heard a
bell and wanted to say to my wife, 'Listen, that's the bell at the
entrance to our cemetery.' But I could not make a sound. I woke up
and felt this extreme cold again and I was absolutely unable to move
or to make a sound. It was a threatening feeling.
However, I had learnt that I did not need to be afraid. And so I
thought to myself, 'Stay calm, you don't need to be afraid. You are
protected.' That made me strong.
Immediately I felt a wave of warmth. This process was already
familiar to me yet it was also a new, deeper experience.
When I was able to think clearly again I thanked God with all my
heart.


## Anxiety

Two weeks later I had one of my regular appointments with my
neurologist. First I told him about my threatening dreams, fear and the
threatening images that appeared suddenly. Today I know that these
were side effects of chemical medications such as antidepressants, which
were the cause of these dreams (see part I, Information leaflets).
The doctor immediately proscribed me lorazepam for my anxiety. I
later read in a daily newspaper that this medication leads to addiction.
This information was already on the information leaflet. I asked
myself, did I come to consultations too infrequently? I insisted on
finding out how I should deal with these night-time events. The
answer I got was, 'That's the ANXIETY, that's what I'm prescribing
you lorazepam for.' So much for detailed information from the doctor.
Clearly I was too bold and annoying with my questions, however,

because upon my insistence at having the required physiotherapy prescribed again, he said that my condition had already improved. He had other patients who needed it more. I did not share this opinion at all and secretly regretted having the audacity to tell the doctor my opinion so directly. That was the end of my physiotherapy prescribed by the doctor.

The topic of anxiety preoccupied me over the following period. Where did this anxiety come from? What was I afraid of?
I learnt during my meditation and when confiding in my physiotherapists that my fear was first and foremost prenatal anxiety. The fear that my mother had experienced due to persecution and rape had probably led to my premature birth.
Anxiety and fear are stress reactions that release stress hormones in the body which spread through the bloodstream. Even babies feel anxiety when they feel alone. This is evident through their crying or an elevated heartbeat. In addition to this, we soon experience anxiety that affects us consciously or unconsciously, triggered, for example, by parents and teachers.
Later in life, politicians, but also doctors, put pressure on us, by categorically rejecting the possibility of natural medicine as an alternative to the pharmaceutical products that are prescribed, for example. Or our employers and bosses use stress to make us open to or even dependent on their goals and commands.

For many of those affected, this anxiety is not only a side effect of medication but is also contributed to by allergies, intolerances, environmental toxins, radiation, amalgam, wood treatment products, etc.
There is then a danger that these anxieties which pile up on top of one another can add up to an all-consuming fear of life which, depending on our constitution, we are no longer able to separate from healthy fears, such as those which are caused by being threatened.

We are only conscious of around 5 to 10 percent of this collection of fears in our nervous system. Physical reactions are the consequence, such as dizziness or sweating (especially at night), feeling hot, internal restlessness, sleep disorders, a racing pulse, unsteadiness when walking, a fear of falling, exhaustion, tiredness, heaviness in the legs, ringing in the ears, feelings of deafness, unexplained pain, etc.
Just like tears when we cry, these reactions are caused by emotional tension, stress, traumatic experiences or conflict with other people. These are clearly signs of fear. It is therefore no wonder that we experience anxiety. A sure way of fighting these fears is not to be alone. It is simply good and comforting to know that there is someone who loves me and is by my side, and helps me to overcome these fears. This someone does not have to be a person. It can also be faith in the god of your belief system, which also gave me security and trust after my terrible dreams.


## Searching

During this year my wife and I wanted to celebrate our fortieth wedding anniversary. We had also recently got a little grandson. If those are not good reasons for self-motivation I am not sure what is!

I definitely wanted to become healthy again! And so I continued searching. And I was surprised by the possibilities.
If not acupuncture, then at least acupressure. As I did not know where the ear meridian is located, I carefully pressed and massaged all over my ears at least twice a day. The burning sensation in my eyes and the tears which cause irritation did not get better. A specialist assured me that it had nothing to do with Parkinson's disease. She could not identify the cause.

## Yoga

The concept of the body, mind and soul as one entity is becoming more and more widely accepted. My wife and I signed up for a yoga course. We were highly sceptical at first and found the course on the sixth floor of a tower block. We were surrounded by a pleasant and relaxed atmosphere. A young woman introduced herself as the leader of the beginners' course. We followed her along with the other participants into a large, light, friendly room. We were the oldest people there and I was the only man. The individual parts of the exercises were first explained in a caring, energetic manner and then demonstrated to us.

We did not stop after this course. Yoga is a wonderful way of experiencing meditation, tension and relaxation. Of course, for Parkinson's sufferers, all of the exercises (known as asanas) are very beneficial. The muscles are addressed directly in equal measure. This means that cramps almost never occur.

As long as the patient does not have high blood pressure, leg exercises and shoulder stands – in particular the plough – are especially effective for Parkinson's sufferers. They directly and efficiently promote blood flow through the brain. Other exercises such as the tree or the crow strengthen the sense of balance. Regardless of which exercises are carried out, the intervals of tension and relaxation benefit the muscles in the entire body.[18]

It is recommended to combine the asanas with treatments that purify the body of acids, heavy metals, fungi and other toxins.

Ever since, an hour of yoga using an exercise CD has been part of our weekly routine. I would no longer want to go without it (see part II, chap. 10, Physiotherapy).

## Healing stones

*God sleeps in stone,*
*breathes in plants,*
*dreams in animals*
*and awakens in people.*
(S. Painadath SJ, India)

Gemstones affect us with their cosmic radiation and vibrations. These
penetrate our deepest layers and influence our wishes and desires, but
also our memories and our health. Healing stones are used all over the
world: in Shamanic traditions, in traditional Chinese medicine (TCM),
in the Indian Ayurveda and in Tibetan medicine. They are used in
almost all natural healing processes.
Gemstone homeopathy, anthroposophic medicine and various other
therapies draw on knowledge of healing stones. These natural
remedies have been known for thousands of years, but are
unfortunately not yet recognised in public as a form of therapy. This
will probably change over the coming years, as it is now possible to
measure the stones' vibrations biophysically. Now people will recognise
what has always worked.

Specialist literature lists the following stones as particularly suitable
for treating Parkinson's disease: emerald, chrysocolla, gold obsidian,
green tourmaline, malachite, mookaite, ryolite, silicon, star sapphire
and chalcedony.[19] The individual healing stone connects and
harmonises the cells through its vibrations. It helps to expand our
consciousness and allow cells to heal. Healing stones are an
important part of the mosaic that makes up the healing process.
For example, the liver has a specific vibration. If it is diseased, I
select the appropriate stone with a similar or higher vibration and
place it on the body to strengthen the liver.
The Swiss biophysicist Walter Stark recognised the lattice vibration
energy of gemstones in the bio-frequency spectrum. The information
from healing stones is absorbed by the approximately 80 billion cells in

the body. If disease is present, they are influenced in such a way as to enable healing. It is now possible to measure the vibrations of healing stones scientifically and/or capture them photographically using biophoton photography. People often buy healing stones based on their appearance or on instinct. From my experience this is not always correct or helpful. Please ask a specialist for advice (see part II, chap. 9, Healing stone therapy; chap, 23. Hildegard therapy).


## Magazines

The 04/2008 issue of the German magazine *Fliege* published an article on Parkinson's disease that was several pages long.[20] The article listed several famous patients and how Parkinson's disease affects them. It contained details of where you can find information and of further treatment such as brain surgery.

What is missing for me is research into the causes.

Where does Parkinson's disease come from? In the media we currently only find poor suggestions or estimates at best. Unfortunately, media articles do not mention any hope of a cure. On the contrary, the lack of a cure for the disease and the need to take medication for the rest of one's life are explicitly mentioned on multiple occasions.

I am fighting against this with all my strength!

Of course, in order to heal we first need information on the cause and *not* the 'magic solution' for the symptoms. Why are patients not at least told about the possibility of natural medicine and spiritual support so that they can make up their own minds?

In the edition of *Fliege* mentioned above I discovered a letter from reader in response to the article which spoke to me so much that I am including the entire text here (translated from the original German):

'Regarding Parkinson's disease, you write that Parkinson's *can* be caused by toxins. Barely any medical experts listen to this. Which toxins are they then? Mainly heavy metals. Certain systems that remove toxins from the body can deal with these well, but others cannot. And this is why we become ill.

When cells contain toxins such as heavy metals, petrochemicals and/or radioactive substances, pesticides, herbicides, etc., they cannot full absorb vitamins and minerals. This causes the disease. The nerves do not get everything they need. Parkinson's disease is big business, this is why no information gets through. But, Mr Fliege, you manage this. It is about the suffering of so many people who have Parkinson's disease, ADHD, autism, etc. It is about all nerve-related diseases. I send you my best wishes!'

So, I must keep looking for the causes in myself. My discoveries might also be able to help other people. I have to find out about the possibilities given to us by nature and our inner divinity.

Just do not give up!

We determine our own lives; the doctor should only be an advisor. Regrettably, however, I increasing have the impression that many people do not want to be helped – after all, applying natural methods consistently over a long period of time is inconvenient. People prefer the quick cocktail of pills from the pharmaceutical industry. And they are proud to be able to say that they now have to take 17 different pills with every meal. People simply do not or do not want to see and evaluate the devastating consequences that this has on the body.

I in no way want to constantly criticise the medical profession. There are certainly situations in which working with a doctor is very beneficial. There are truly some fantastic surgeons, heart specialists, etc. However, in my opinion, starting during medical training, there is unfortunately a failure to see the person as a whole and to concentrate on the causes of disease.

Many doctors do not seem at all willing to do this. Why not though? Many undergo further training to learn about diseases in detail.

I believe that doctors have one of two different hearts beating in their chests. Some have a heart for patients and genuinely want to help them without considering any negative consequences from the health insurance providers. However, the other kind of heart wants to use the newest magic pills every two weeks to keep the pharmaceutical reps happy...

Luckily I have usually encountered doctors who have a heart for me and have not hesitated to help me, sometimes giving me free examinations.
This must also be stated clearly for the record! I would like to take this opportunity to say a huge, genuine thank you to these incredibly caring people and true helpers.

There really are many doctors who selflessly prove every day that they want to help patients. My criticism is only aimed at the few but drastic examples of this profession who do not shy away from treating a patient purely on the basis of costs.
Luckily there are also other doctors, such as Dr Manfred Jucho. A quotation from the July edition of *Fliege* (translated from German): 'Healing is always a blessing! And is about taking it.'[20]
The German magazine *Welt der Wunder* (issue 3/2008) published another extraordinary article about how music heals the brain[21].
Music therapy for people with brain damage is a wonderful opportunity to make movement smoother without any damaging side effects. In the article, Oliver Sacks reports that music works like a pacemaker from the outside, because music affects wide areas of the brain. In July 2008, the German television channel ZDF presented several Parkinson's sufferers in an episode of its programme *38 Grad*.[22]
While such articles and programmes are an important way of creating awareness of Parkinson's disease, I feel there is a serious lack of research into the cause and information on how the disease develops. All of the Parkinson's sufferers in the television programme had worked in management positions and been under a great deal of stress.
Why are the actual causes not mentioned? Because people do not want to see them?

## Natural medicine at German universities

My psychotherapist, who I trust greatly, gave me a tip about a particular university hospital. I sent a message asking for help. I received an answer the very same day.
I thought that was fantastic.

Professor A, a professor of natural medicine at the hospital, wrote to me saying that he was about to go on holiday for the semester break. He suggested that it was best to contact the university's expert on Parkinson's disease.
The next day I was lucky enough to be put into contact with the Parkinson's specialist Professor B immediately. We had a very pleasant discussion, during which he did not rush and explained to me his position and the situation in his department. He said directly that he did not work with natural medicine. He was a surgeon. At the university hospital, under his direction, Parkinson's patients had the 'brain chips' that are talked about in the media implanted. According to him, it is a simple and relatively risk-free operation.
From the way he said it I believed it too. He asked me what medication I was taking. In his opinion, I could still wait a while before having surgery. He said that this was always done as a last resort in order to drastically reduce the amount of medication needed. This was also probably very successful.

This might be an option for Parkinson's sufferers in whom the disease is very advanced and for whom the natural therapies no longer offer sufficient, quick success. However, the natural therapies should definitely be used as a complementary treatment to limit the side effects of the medication to a bearable level.

After I asked again about the possibility of natural therapies he
referred me back to Professor A mentioned above, the natural medicine
specialist at the university hospital. I wrote him another e-mail asking
him to help me in my search for the causes of Parkinson's disease and
the possibility of natural healing.

In November 2009, Professor B gave a comprehensive explanation of
the possibility of a surgical implant in a television programme. This
was a good occasion to ask again about the most up-to-date
information. In his reply he told me that the professor of natural
medicine was unable to help me as it was not his area of
specialisation.
At the same time I contacted the university hospital in Berlin. A new
institute with a young professor of natural medicine had just been
set up there. Unfortunately I never received a reply to my letter or
e-mails.
So much for natural medicine at German universities.
Maybe my questions were not expressed scientifically enough. After
all, I'm just a sick man looking for help.


## Special case PSP

Through intensive discussions and e-mail exchanges with other
sufferers I learnt about PSP.
PSP – progressive supranuclear palsy, also known as Steele-
Richardson-Olszewski syndrome after the doctors who discovered it –
is a disease which is very similar to Parkinson's disease but is
unknown to may surgeons and therefore often goes untreated.
As with Parkinson's disease, PSP suffers have limited movement
(bradykinesia). Muscle stiffness (rigor) is particularly severe in the neck
and torso. Resting tremor is also present, as in Parkinson's disease, but is
less frequent.
However, a grave difference is the eye movement disorder. PSP sufferers
cannot lower the gaze, i.e. they cannot look down. This disorder is typical

of PSP. Sight problems such as double or blurred vision can be signs of PSP. When they fall, patients usually fall backwards.

It has been discovered that a protein (the tau protein which produces microtubules) is formed in the nerve cells but also the nerve cells' supporting tissue (the astroglia), similarly to what happens in patients with Alzheimer's disease.

It is suspected that this is caused by a virus which has been in the body for years or even decades. Another possible cause is a genetic mutation in brain cells. A reaction between free radicals and important components of the cells causes damage to the cells which can lead to PSP. A further possible cause is poisoning which, for example, has been observed on the islands of Guam and Guadeloupe. PSP, Parkinson's disease and Alzheimer's disease are common there.

If you suspect PSP, please seek detailed information and speak to your neurologist.


## Magnetism

The August edition of the magazine *Welt der Wunder* published another report which discussed possible future treatments for Alzheimer's disease and other brain diseases.[23]

The topic of the article was how the secret powers of magnetism work, and it discussed, for example, the possibilities of TMS (transcranial magnet stimulation) as a promising treatment for impairment of cerebral function.

Natural electrical currents in the heart, kidney and other organs create a magnetic field in the human body. The brain is also a 'magnetic organ'. Researchers aim to deliver nerve impulses which pass on signals in order to transmit information in the brain via electrical processes on the cell membranes. These processes are controlled with magnetic fields which are 1000 times stronger than the Earth's magnetic field, but the impulses last only a thousandth of a second.

This means that TMS could be used to accompany learning processes and make healthy parts of the brain take on the functions of the damaged regions. The researchers are also interested in the possibilities of TMS for short-term stimulation in savant syndrome.

Can magnetic fields boost IQ? There must be something to this because, as with all good discoveries, the military have expressed interest in the development.
The United States Department of Defense wants to use this technique to disable parts of the brain for a certain period of time in order to 'turn off' fatigue and tiredness in soldiers who are on continuous operations or in conflict zones.


## Active ingredients

In September, in a programme called *Fakt,* the German television channel ARD reported on the contracts for enormous discounts that the pharmaceutical industry gives health insurance providers by providing substitute medications.[24]

Recently, rather than being given a prescription for a particular medication, some patients have been receiving prescriptions that simply state an active ingredient. This means that the patient is given a medication by the pharmacy for which their doctor does not know the side effects because they only prescribe the active ingredient.
The frightening effect of this substitution of medications is that the patient may go to a different pharmacy after each visit to the doctor and may therefore be given different medications which have the same active ingredient but could have different side effects.
The patient then has to deal with stomach pains, headaches, and kidney or bowel problems.
The medications that were discussed in the report were particularly important for diseases such as high blood pressure, diabetes, Parkinson's disease and epilepsy.

Here it seems that patients are once again being used a guinea pigs. Yet we trust the doctor and still believe that they know the medications prescribed to cure us inside out. However, what do we usually hear when we complain about painful side effects? 'You'll have to live with that now.'

No thank you, medication must work precisely!

## Meals on wheels

Many people rely on meals on wheels due to illness or old age. This also applies to many Parkinson's patients. These meals are often manufactured for these consumers by industrial companies. The German Nutrition Society believes that these meals should be particularly nutritious and rich in vitamins and minerals, and must have a high nutrient density. Unfortunately the opposite is often true. Using various sample meals, it was discovered that the meals do not meet expectations, neither visually nor in terms of their content. The meals offered should contain an average of 33 mg of vitamin C and 3 µg (microgrammes) of vitamin D. Both values in the sample meals were 0. It was a similar story with minerals. The following should be present: 333 mg calcium, 117 mg magnesium and 133 mg folic acid, which is particularly important for older people. The manufacturers of the food did put in 56 mg of magnesium. 'Better than nothing' is no consolation here. Keep in mind that the customers are not able to get other food themselves. How should our metabolism and immune systems be stabilised if not, first and foremost, through nutrition? It must not simply be about filling our stomachs; food must help us to become healthy again. Is that a utopian idea?[25]

## Nanoparticles

A new series of articles discussed the use of nanoparticles. These nanoparticles, loaded with effective medications, are released into the blood to activate a targeted boost to healing in the body. This method is used today against cancers and brain tumours, for example.[26]

A nanoparticle is one millionth of a millimetre in size. The worrying thing is that the food industry already adds nanoparticles to over 600 different products, for example, as an anti-caking agent for sugar and salt.

The amounts of these nanoparticles that are added are more or less uncontrolled, as in Germany and most other countries there are still no regulations concerning their use. Tiny aluminium particles are added to junk food, silicon dioxide is in ketchup and sauces, titanium dioxide is found in chocolate and chocolate-based products... The list goes on.

There is no end in sight. In a way which is completely uncontrolled and sometimes without any indication or warnings, our bodies are forced to process these industrial additives on a day to day basis. Are they capable of this?

Critics and researchers say no, because the smaller the particles of a substance are, the larger their surface area in relation to their volume. Inflammation and damage to our cells' DNA – this is what they are talking about. Yet no one wants to know exactly what amounts of nanoparticles endanger our bodies' health.[27]

We have barely any knowledge or confirmation of the dangers. The food industry keeps pressing forward. If it is proven that they cause damage, the parent company or the affiliates in the pharmaceutical industry will no doubt develop a suitable medication for it.

Can we protect ourselves against nanoparticles? Only by eating natural organic food and freshly prepared organic products. If we only eat food from the mainstream food industry we have no way of protecting ourselves.

## Dowsing

I finally had the necessary information and the opportunity to measure and correct the geopathic values in my house. This applied particularly to where I slept.

You know the feeling of sleeping restlessly, waking up drenched in sweat and feeling exhausted the next day? Whenever I spent a day at home I often felt strangely and worryingly uneasy. After my experiences from the previous year measuring my food and the things around me with the pendulum, I was anxious to finally measure the rooms where I slept and worked too.

Several years before, I had had the opportunity to go looking for water with a dowser. The aim then was to find a good source for a well on a friend's property. I was already fascinated then by the possibility of finding where and how deep water was based on the closing of the metal rods, as well as knowing how many litres of water per minute were to be expected.

It caught my interest and I wanted to try it for myself now.

Using my pendulum I had already found out more or less where the concerning areas were in and around my house, which provided an explanation for my restlessness. These were around my bed, my dining table and my desk. However, other areas that I did not spend so much time in were also affected.

I got the dowsing rod from my friend who had used the dowser on his property. This dowser was a professor of geophysics at a university in the Ruhr area in Germany.

I simply copied how he had held the dowsing rod. It worked immediately. When my wife tried dowsing, on the other hand, there was no reaction.

A floor plan of the building helped us to see exactly where the water went in and out underneath the building. This enabled us to find seven water veins underneath the house.

This was not surprising as our house is located in a heavily wooded area on the side of a hill. Hurricane Kyrill had blown the trees down, meaning that the wood was almost completely gone and rain water now flowed down the hill unused. When we connected where the inflow and outflow of water was based on the floor plan, we were able to locate the cross-over points fairly exactly, with a few small deviations as water does not flow completely straight. It did not surprise me that they were exactly in the places where I had already detected damaging energy using the pendulum.

Dear reader, this section is not intended to turn you into a dowser. Simply knowing where water flows is of course not enough. There is more to it, including information about earth grid systems, as Dr Ernst Hartmann, Dr Manfred Curry and many others have found out. That would be going into too much detail here, but it is important to me to make you aware of the possibilities of finding out the causes for your disease.

If you believe that water veins or other geopathic anomalies cannot be ruled out as a cause, I recommend that you consult a trained specialist in geopathy, geobiology or geophysics, as the influences of geological energy such as earth radiation, water veins or Hartmann grids are very much able to cause diseases such as cancer, Parkinson's, MS and tachycardia. These diseases often begin with many years of sleeplessness.
Anyone who believes that earth radiation only affects people who live on the ground floor is mistaken. Measurements show that on the third floor, for example, earth radiation is much stronger than on the ground floor of a house. Piping for water and sewage, as well as electrical cabling and antennae, which sometimes run around the walls, allow for earth radiation to increase in strength in a spiralling manner. Earth radiation can even have a crucial effect on couples who are unable to have children.

Geopathy (geo = earth; pathogen = causing disease) researches the geopathical stress zones that can cause illness. The term 'geopathy' was coined by Professor Johann Walther, a geologist and palaeontologist at the University of Halle in Germany, in the 1920s. In the 19030s, the French doctor Dr F. R. Peyré described a global grid starting from the north pole with squares with four-metre-long sides which, according to his research, had considerable effect on people's health.

Gustav Freiherr von Pohl was the first to discover a correlation between the results of dowsing and the development of disease. In 1930, he reported on his research for the first time at a doctors' congress in Munich. In July 1930, he wrote an article for the Berlin-based cancer research magazine *Krebsforschung* about the development of cancers due to earth currents. His book *Earth Currents: Causative Factor of Cancer and Other Diseases* was published in 1932. Following on from the comprehensive work by Dr Ernst Hartmann in 1967 entitled *Krankheit als Standortproblem* (illness as a disease of location), working groups for building biology were set up in Belgium, the Netherlands, Austria and Switzerland in the 1970s and 80s. The currents found in the locations where MS and cancer patients lived provided information about the typical constellations of stress zones. For example:

Intersection of two geomantic zones
Intersection of the main zones of several water veins
Intersection of congruent zones of different grids
Horizontal zone of the first and second grid at the height at which the bed lies

The results of current research bring this information out of the fog of belief and enable them to be measured physically. Help is possible, as since these discoveries have been made research has also focused on finding ways of shielding us from these areas which cause disease. In this context, it is important to draw attention to the fact that patients with multiple sclerosis, Alzheimer's disease and Parkinson's

disease may show the same damage in different areas of the brain, nerves and musculature. It therefore cannot be ruled out that the causes of these diseases may be geopathic.
There are some natural and very inexpensive methods of counteracting harmful currents. Seek expert advice. Particularly with regard to the places where one sleeps, eats and works, it may be that your bed or desk can simply be moved to another location. This is often sufficient. Unfortunately, this is not always the case.[28]


## Side Effects: Death

The book *Side Effects: Death*[29] by John Virapen gives a clear and blunt description of the doings of the pharmaceutical industry. Many of the chapters are about Prozac, which contains the active ingredient fluoxetine that is also licenced for use in Germany. When the licencing application was submitted, Prozac was initially judged too dangerous. Later, however, the person responsible for processing the application at the German department of health no longer considered it dangerous and approved the product for sale.
Mr Virapen worked as a manager at a pharmaceutical giant himself and knew what he was talking about when he described certain medications in detail.
His book is about the poorly adapted child ADHD sufferers who had to take these products containing fluoxetine – a medication that makes people world-weary and aggressive. Virapen also addresses many other medications on the market, discussing their origins, active ingredients, and effects, how they were developed and the process of licensing with the authorities. In this context, it is irrelevant what the medication is called, what matters in terms of its effects is the active ingredient. Fluoxetine was contained in the medications that I was prescribed for years.
Quote:

`**Fluoxetine**. The name of an active ingredient. The product names
are *Prozac*® (USA, Great Britain) *Fluctin*® (Germany) and *Fluctine*®
(Switzerland, Austria). Fluoxetin belongs to the family of SSRIs. It is
used to treat depression, obsessive-compulsive disorders and bulimia.
Suicide is one of the side effects. The use of this antidepressant in
children and adolescents, except for improved indications, is extremely
dangerous. In this combination, suicidal behaviour (suicidal thoughts,
and suicide attempts), as well as hostility (predominantly aggression,
oppositional behaviour and anger) were observed in clinical trials. This
is valid for all medications in the SSRI group.'[30]

I will now refer back to the early stages of my Parkinson's disease
from 2003 to 2006. During this time, neurologists kept giving me
tablets with the active ingredient fluoxetine. Now I see this as the
explanation for the dark, unhealthy thoughts about death that I
had at the time.
As I kept the information sheets and instructions for use that came
with the medication, this research is actually the simplest.
Essentially, the side effects of these three pharmaceutical products
which cause illness are indeed very similar. Here are some short
summaries:

### Medication: Fluoxetin beta® 40

Active ingredient: fluoxetine hydrochloride, equivalent to 40mg of
fluoxetine
Which side effects can occur when taking Fluoxetin beta® 40?
Dry mouth, complaints of the central nervous system such as
headaches, anxiety, shaking, nightmares, restlessness, liver function
disorders of varying severity; extrapyramidal symptoms (movement
disorders) may be especially likely to occur in patients with a pre-
existing condition (e.g. Parkinson's disease); additionally suicidal
thoughts, aggressive behaviour, etc.

**Medication: Fluneurin® 40mg tabs**

Active ingredient: fluoxetine hydrochloride
Which side effects can occur when taking Fluneurin® 40 mg tabs?
Anxiety, thought disorder, pain in the arms and legs;
extrapyramidal symptoms (movement disorders) may be especially
likely to occur or worsen in patients with a pre-existing condition
(e.g. Parkinson's disease); additionally gastrointestinal bleeding,
aggressive behaviour, etc.

**Medication: Fluoxetin-neuraxpharm® 20 T**

Active ingredient: fluoxetine hydrochloride, 22.4 mg per tablet
Which side effects can occur when taking Fluoxetin-neurax-pharm® 20 T?
Nervousness, restlessness, sleep disorders, unusual dreams, impaired
vision, confusion, aggression, states of unrest, depression, suicidal
thoughts, loss of ability to concentrate, etc.

On these incredibly long information sheets I see many specialist
medical terms which are not comprehensible to a layperson without a
medical dictionary. I think that these small, shortened lists which use
more general terms are sufficient in order to recognise how these
chemical preparations make people 'healthy' again.

Especially now, as I am writing these things down, it becomes clear
to me how important my new way of looking at things has become
– moving away from chemical medications to natural medications
without side effects.

## Aronia melanocarpa/aronia berries

In West Germany, the otherwise largely unknown aronia berry has
been known as a powerful antioxidant for over 100 years. Originally
from the east of North America, they came to Russia around the year
1900. There the fruit was grown by the now famous fruit grower
Mitschurin. A trial plantation with over 20 000 shrubs was planted in
St Petersburg.

In former East Germany, the aronia berries were first grown around 1976 in the agricultural cooperative *Berglandobst*. Aronia berries were also planted and processed successfully in Slovakia and Scandinavia, a blessing for natural medicine. From there they spread across Europe. More than 50 years ago, the first indications of their healing effects became apparent in the former Soviet Union.
Aronia berries have a significant role to play in the healing of various lifestyle diseases. German universities have shown the positive effect of aronia berries on the following diseases: Parkinson's disease, Alzheimer's disease, multiple sclerosis, psoriasis, rheumatism, age-related macular degeneration, asthma, chronic bronchitis, inflammatory bowel diseases, diabetes, hepatitis, cancer, and many more.

No other food has such a high level of anti-oxidant anthocyanins as the aronia berry. Anthocyanins keep the proportion of free radicals and anti-oxidants balanced so that we can stay healthy. Drinking fresh aronia juice once or twice daily for two to three weeks is also a natural method of reducing blood pressure. Aronia berries are a fantastic natural medicine for bronchitis, especially for children. During pregnancy they are thought to have highly beneficial effects on the mother and the growth of the baby.[31]

I have had an aronia shrub in my garden since 2007. I will have to wait a few more years before it begins to flower and bear fruit.
Nature has everything ready for us; we just need to take it. It is very simple! I can think of a short story in relation to this: A good friend and lover of home-grown fruit and vegetables only cautiously decided, when she was 50 years old, to start eating black-coloured berries such as blueberries, blackcurrants and blackberries. She was brought up this way. Her mother had taught all of her children what the priest had said from the pulpit: 'All black berries come from the devil! You must not eat them!'

So much for a sensible approach to what are actually incredibly healthy black fruits and vegetables offered by nature.


## Healing with energy

Towards the end of the year I was asked at a seminar how I had found out about various possible treatments for Parkinson's disease. I tried to explain that I had not found or discovered or identified these treatments, or however you want to put it. They were given to me. After my urgent prayer a few years previously I had felt that I was being guided. I was guided to places and information and people that could help me to beat my disease.
This experience taught me that we all carry a great amount of God's power of self-healing in ourselves.
We can activate it!

We are human beings. We were taught the Latin words of humanism at school. These are associated with humanity; how humans should interact with one another. However, it is not widely known that the word 'human' does not come from Latin at all but is a Sanskrit term, many centuries old:
*Hu* means light. *Man* means being.[32]
From the being of creation, we humans were designed to be 'light beings'. As light beings, we have large amounts of energy as an expression of our possibilities, be they for healing or everyday things. A wise script describes this as follows: 'God, I am fully able to succeed in all my endeavours that I start truthfully.'[33]

Over the coming decades, I hope, people will learn more and more about how this power can serve human wellbeing. The medicine of the future will stem from universal power and energy by making use of the teachings of quantum physics.
After all, today it is a scientific fact that everything is energy. Every material, and every non-material, everybody, every plant, every

stone, the air that we breathe, water, feelings, thoughts – all of these are made up of measurable energy. This is measured in nanometres, which are millionths of metres.

This energy benefits people. It renews the more than 80 billion cells in our bodies, renews our health – the health of every person, every animal, every plant, *everywhere*! We must simply be ready and learn to ask and give thanks for it.

It is very simple.

And how are our personal energy levels, our vibrations, today, at this moment? Let us start by surrounding ourselves with things that have a high level of energy.

Let us start by ensuring that the things we eat and drink have high levels of energy. Our bread, our water, vegetables, fruit, whatever it may be – look for them and you will receive the things that are right for you. Maybe not immediately and directly; you have to work on it, but with time you will feel it yourself. Your body will yearn to only consume these high-quality things (in terms of energy) to gladly gain more and more knowledge and experience, and also to make distinctions.

With conscious living we are able over time to better perceive and recognise the things we consume – what is good and right, and what we would do better to refuse.

The power of the universe is rooted deep within us, because we are part of the universe. We have the power and the ability to take in energy and pass it on – to people, animals and plants.


## Elementary meditation

This programme focuses on a holistic approach to the relationship between body, mind and soul. It is based on activating our chakras, the energy centres of our bodies. Activating our chakras allows us to use elementary energy effectively and transfer it to ourselves and other people.

The pure love that comes from the heart is shaped by human beings' compassion and helpfulness for all living things in this world. During my daily meditation I try to comprehend the magnificence of this. I am always surprised how I am guided further and further. First I am led in my thoughts to the people close to me – my family, my friends – and later to my possibility of being able to transfer energy to all living things. It is a wonderful feeling for me to be able to pass on this immense knowledge in my seminars today.
I remember my prayer from two years ago. The final sentence was 'Love and compassion should fill me'. Back then I knew nothing of the possibilities of elementary meditation and transferring energy. It is wonderful!
THANK YOU for this year that has brought me so far.


## 2009 – Powers of self-healing through natural therapies


I felt a new vitality emerging, but I was pushed to my limits again and again on a daily basis.
I got my sense of fun back.
Sometimes I thought that I was getting my old wit back.
Slowly my mental capacities came back and not only could I read the newspaper, I could understand it again.
At my wife's suggestion I began a kind of memory therapy. I started to write down my experiences with the doctors and with medicine to record the valuable knowledge I had gained regarding natural healing powers, as well as my own chances of healing, so that I could make it available to other people with the same problems. It would be fantastic if I were able to help many of those affected in this way. I wanted this with all my heart.

## Powers of self-healing

The French pharmacist Emil Coué lived at the end of the 19th century and said one specific thing that made him world-famous at the time: 'To fear a disease is to cause it!'
When I really think about this, I see that it is true. Whether we ourselves or one of our friends say, 'I always get a bad back in this weather,' then we end up having it shortly afterwards. I want to learn to think differently. I will simply change my thoughts. Our consciousness can be changed easily and quickly. To stay with my previous example, I could say, 'I am well, my back is strong and powerful!' All of the positive thoughts are contained in this sentence – it is not difficult. Once we are able to ignore the educational values we have been taught by our parents, teachers and superiors, it can work. This takes time, but overcoming this bad habit of always thinking the worst that is ingrained in us is a truly beneficial experience with life-long effects. Another sentence secured Coué true world-wide fame: *Tous les jours à tous points de vue je vais de mieux en mieux!*
This means: Every day I get better and better in every respect![34]
This is my new motto; it is exactly how I feel about my new life.


## Detoxification instead of toxification

A friend of mine gave me a book by the alternative practitioner Uwe Karstädt entitled *Entgiften statt vergiften* (detoxification instead of toxification). I highly recommend it. It documents in clear, direct language the negative effects of food, medications and similar products in our society.[35] This makes it very informative for laypeople as well. Karstädt finds many indications of the negative effects of industrially-produced food and of our environment.
For example, he describes the relationship between Alzheimer's disease and the toxic effects of aluminium on the body. He also describes this in relation to other diseases, such as anaemia, muscle pain, osteoporosis, inflammation of the large intestine, kidney inflammation, kidney dysfunction, liver disease, stomach complaints,

stomach ulcers, hyperactivity, ADD, constipation, headaches, heartburn and more.

Uwe Karstädt writes about the toxic metal manganese and its effects, such as emotional instability, muscle weakness, headaches, balance problems, dementia, tiredness, violence, 'manganese insanity', lack of dopamine, Parkinson's disease, tremors, lack of facial expression and more.

In this brilliant book of advice he of course mentions other toxic metals which cause illness, but it was those given above that resonated most with me. The symptoms matched those that I was dealing with exactly.


## Iris diagnosis

At a visit to conference in Baden-Baden with over 120 expert presentations we met an alternative practitioner who worked with iris diagnosis. He had never seen me before. After diagnosis using my iris he explained the problems with my brain, my liver, etc. to me. I was impressed. When I told him about my Parkinson's problems he gave me some additional advice. I should start oxygen therapy at home to provide my brain with sufficient oxygen. He also advised me to have lymph drainage therapy from a good physiotherapist until I was able to perform it myself.

Over these few days my wife and I also met several specialists who worked with healing stones. We had been looking for such people for a long time. A very nice woman suggested my wife buy the book *Health through God's Pharmacy*[36]. In this book I found additional information on what grows in herbs gardens and can be used to fight Parkinson's disease. In a psychotherapy session with a professor in Dusseldorf I was given another fantastic piece of advice. To my surprise, he said something very open-minded that is not often heard from doctors: 'Anyone who heals is right.' His advice encouraged me to investigate craniosacral therapy. The term did not mean much to me then. However, when I went to my Aslan therapy the next day and saw a poster on the front door advertising a presentation about craniosacral therapy in the seminar room at four o'clock, I was once again surprised to experience such a 'coincidence'. In actual fact I would no longer have needed it but it was still fascinating to see once again how simple things can be when you are guided.


## Aslan therapy

It all started with me needing to go for a stay at a medical spa again. Due to my rheumatic diseases I had being gathering experience with moor baths since I was 16 years old. I had been travelling to Upper Bavaria for these baths for over 30 years and was always very pleased with the effects.
My wife thought that we should try something new – close by without the need for long journeys.
We had heard of the Aslan Institute that offered spa therapy for general stabilisation of the body, such as by preventing signs of ageing and strengthening the immune system. These treatments were developed back in the 1960s by Professor Ana Aslan.
Professor Aslan was born in Romania in 1897. During treatment in Romanian hospitals she discovered that the active ingredient procaine that had previously only been used as an anaesthetic made the body fitter and more powerful in very small doses. She used this as a basis for treatment concepts designed to combat wear and ageing processes, with international success. This was the state of my knowledge when I went for my treatment.

We were met with a pleasant atmosphere. Very friendly staff and caring nurses greeted us and explained the process to us. Then we had an initial conversation with the doctor who ran the institute. There were many more to come, which were carried out with a thoroughness that we had not experienced before, with comprehensive questions and intense discussions that lasted almost two hours.

Over the following three weeks I was give procaine injections every day, including on Saturdays and Sundays, which were enriched with vitamins, minerals and trace elements mixed individually according to my current state and the doctor's diagnosis, a new combination almost every day.
What other doctor takes care of their patients over the entire course of treatment and is available to talk every day? The doctors at my previous medical spa treatment courses were not. They were only there for me once a week. This was an entirely new, very positive experience! Furthermore, I was given physiotherapy by a skilled team whose cheerfulness was contagious. As I had already had over 10 years of experience with physiotherapy I know what I am talking about. I felt very at ease and very safe. The exercises pushed me to my limits but I was able to trust them. Even unpleasant treatment like lymph drainage on my head and around my mouth was bearable because of this.
Cheerfulness and skill are the best strategies when working with patients. Ozone and light therapy, ultrasound therapy, Nordic walking, a quartz sand treatment table, two hours of yoga a week, a variety of presentations by doctors and more meant that time went by very quickly. During our final discussion the doctor in charge gave me copies of the first publications by Professor Aslan from the 1960s about procaine for Parkinson's patients. I was especially pleased by this and it was helpful for my continuing research into holistic methods of healing.

During the treatment I felt good but not better. However, that soon changed. Two to three weeks later I already felt that something was changing in me. I felt much better, stronger, and I suddenly trusted myself to do to a great number of things when I would have previously said, 'Leave me at home, I just want some peace and quiet.'

This treatment concept is a form of holistic medicine. It contains conventional and alternative treatments; the daily procaine injections or infusions and the physiotherapy that is tailored to the needs of each patient, in combination with magnetic field and oxygen therapy, etc. This was simply very effective for me.


## Craniosacral therapy

The head of the physiotherapy department at the Aslan Institute was a specialist in the craniosacral therapy that I had been made aware of.
First I went to the introductory presentation. It was very interesting.

It has been known in medicine for a reasonably long time that there is a liquid, the cerebrospinal fluid, that surrounds the brain and spinal cord and is produced by the meninges.
However, the knowledge that this fluid moves rhythmically – in a way that is distinct from the heartbeat, i.e. the cardiovascular system – is relatively new.
The term 'cranio' comes from Greek and means head; 'sacral' refers to the sacrum, the bone at the base of the spine.
The craniosacral system works with the knowledge that the skull bones of a healthy adult are not connected firmly and fused together, as is often claimed. At what are known as the seams, movements between the cranial bones are possible. By moving the individual cranial bones slightly the meninges and cerebrospinal fluid are stimulated.
The job of the craniosacral therapist is to activate and stimulate the rhythmic flow of the fluid from the base of the spine to the skull. The therapist activates the fluid so that it can flow unhindered up the spinal tracts to the head, where it can flow around the brain.
Craniosacral therapy is a form of treatment that was passed on by the Shawnee Native Americans. The first person to write about it

was Andrew Taylor Still (1828–1917). It was developed into its current form by Dr John Upledger, who runs an institute offering this therapy in America. He gives lectures on the subject all over the world.[37]

Textbooks and reference books on the therapy have been published in Italy since the 1920s. Unfortunately, in Germany it is still largely unknown.

The even, pulsating flow of the fluid in the body shows the therapist how healthy the patient is and what type of diseases they have. They are also able to feel any disruptions that have a negative effect on the body and wellbeing as a whole and to treat them.

What causes disruptions in the pulsating rhythm? Falls or blows or similar accidents are often the cause, sometimes those which happened during our early childhood. The flow of liquid in the spinal tract from the sacrum to the head may also be disrupted by operations, for example operations on the spine.

At universities in Germany it is common knowledge that this fluid exists, but the fact that the fluid has its own pulse has not yet found its way into teaching and research across the country.

Craniosacral therapists need to be very sensitive in order to feel the state of the body. Experienced therapists work with the knowledge that tissue has a kind of memory. Just as the brain stores memories and experiences, our organs and tissue are also able to do so.

This is entering the domain of psychology when old incidents, known as trauma or energy blockages are re-experienced by the body. Under the effects of the mild heat that is produced during the therapy, the blockages are gently levelled out. In this way, craniosacral therapy works with the 'inner doctor', the inner knowledge of things that have happened to us – but, thank God, also with the inner knowledge that we can heal ourselves again. A good therapist is 'merely' a guide who knows about of powers of self-healing.

This way of working with energy has a general healing effect. The range of applications for craniosacral therapy is as astounding as it is broad, just like the system itself.
Here are a few examples:
Infections, sprains, bruises, strains, etc.
Chronic pain, arthritis, emotional problems, scoliosis, ear problems, minor strokes, visual problems, headaches, back pain, multiple sclerosis, brain damage, nerve damage, coma patients, etc.
Pregnancy and obstetrics, help for new-borns and infants, all childhood diseases, ADD/ADHD, Down's syndrome, epileptic fits, learning difficulties, etc.

I began craniosacral treatment as part of my Aslan therapy and can say that it only improved my health. However, I was very lucky to have found an incredibly good therapist.

*Please note:* Of course, the case here is again that therapies that really help are not covered by statutory health insurance providers in Germany. I cannot help feeling that this system is fighting on the side of disease.
Erich Fromm summed this up so accurately:
A healthy economy is only possible at the expense of unhealthy human beings.


## Maria Treben

I finally bought Maria Treben's book *Health through God's Pharmacy*. I was overwhelmed by the number of different healing techniques suggested for the most diverse of diseases. Among other things, the book said that the tremor in Parkinson's disease could be eased and possibly even healed with wood sorrel. [38]
For the brain Maria Treben suggests compresses on the back of the head with the Swedish bitters that she has tried for various purposes. I tried this after reading about it and have been using the

compresses at home when I am alone ever since. You can feel it
stimulating the scalp and the regions below.
I consider these compresses very helpful as long as you get used to
the constant smell of alcohol. I did not always find this easy. In the
long term I could feel a noticeable release of tension in the affected
region of my brain, and that was what counted in the end.
It is good to see that there are resources given to us by nature that
can have a healing influence, even without scientific evidence.


## Sonntags-Blick

In an edition of the Swiss newspaper *Sonntags-Blick* from  15
February 2009 I found an important article related to Parkinson's
disease. The subject of the article was pesticides and bee mortality.
The article noted that contact with pesticides increases the risk of
Parkinson's disease by 70 percent. Substances used to kill insects
are particularly dangerous.
Dr Fabio Baronti is an expert on Parkinson's disease at Bethesda Klinik
in Tschugg near Bern. He believes certain pesticides cannot be ruled
out as a contributing factor in Parkinson's disease. Later in the article
he mentions clothianidin, an insecticide that is used on maize, among
other plants.
In the Upper Rhine region alone it is thought that 12,000 of Germany's
bee colonies have been poisoned by it. The manufacturer, a large
German chemical producer, provided the bee keepers with
compensation. In Switzerland too, a third of all bee colonies died
between 2005 and 2008. This insecticide has been banned in France
and Canada for many years. Based on a study by Professor Girolami a
ban has also been in place in Germany and Italy since 2009.
Parkinson's is a disease that results from the sum of different
stresses experienced over many years. For these reason, even if the
disease develops later, it is worth checking what contact the sufferer
has had with insecticides, pesticides and similar toxins.

On 27 February 2009, I discovered a report on *SPIEGEL Online* with the title 'Verdrängter Schrecken' (suppressed terror).

It was about the experiences that hundreds of thousands of people suffered during the war, but also in the following few years, due to expulsion or famine. [39]

Whether this was as an infant or child or in the womb makes no difference. The events, the shock, the hunger and the fear cannot be erased. They deeply concern those affected; the neuropsychological processes are still active in the present day.

The older we get, the more the experiences – our own or our mothers' – affect us in the form of fear and anxiety. This fear and anxiety can manifest itself as, for example, depression, cramps, an elevated heartrate or even chronic pain. Even people who did not experience the war themselves still feel unresolved feelings of loss and deficiency within themselves.

Geneticists have discovered through studies that these traumatic experiences can even change our genes and that children and these children's children can still suffer because of them. At the time I was not aware of my mother's terrible situation which led to me being born prematurely and the living conditions after my birth, but I still stored these experiences within myself.

When I was two years old my father returned from the prisoner of war camp and saw me for the first time. My parents then decided to move from Allgäu back to the Ruhr area with my older sister and me. They managed it somehow, travelling through various occupied zones on some of the few remaining functioning trains.

This journey took a week, in carriages without windows or seats, in ice-cold train stations and waiting rooms, with constant disruptions due to damaged tracks and bombed cities. Apart from a little corn flour we had nothing to eat.

Our generation must learn to deal with what we have experienced and to talk about it, as difficult as it can be. Only by doing so will we be able to overcome it and become freer.

## Peace and quiet

Sometimes I just wanted my peace and quiet. I wanted things
around me to be quiet; no roads, aeroplanes, building sites or
anything like that. I wanted an inner peace. I had a kind of longing
for quiet. I was happy when I had the opportunity to experience
this.
To simply sit still.
This loud world was making me ill.
Today I know that quietness can heal.
The peace that I feel when I have gone inside myself for a few
minutes is the true centre of my existence. To look for this peace in
prayer, alone in a church, in the woods, or on a bench at the side of
a path, makes it easy for me. All religions in this world are based on
similar mystical experiences – when the brain's activity is switched
off by peace and quiet.
Our minds often see this differently. They think that one thing or
another is more important in this moment. But our minds often lie
to us, as they only tell us the things that we allow them to store
over the course of our lives.
When our bodies feel this strong need for quiet, we should give
them a chance to rest. Unfortunately, in most cases we need to
practice this before we are able to do so.
Of course, there are courses and instructions for this. But why not
just try it for yourself?
Make sure you are sitting comfortably in a chair and that any possible
sources of interruption, such as doorbells and telephones, are turned
off. Take a deep breath in and out at least three times and try to let
your mind become still.
Say a few affirmations to yourself, such as:
'Peace and quiet are flowing through my body'.
You can repeat this several times like a mantra or say a prayer; if
you find it helpful it could be one from your childhood. Simply go
with what you know and trust. You should try to become 'empty' in
order to feel peace with all of your senses.

You have to leave the everyday world outside. Over time you will succeed if you truly want to.

Please take at least 10 to 20 minutes every day for these exercises. You can start your day with them or integrate them into your daily routine. The most important thing is that you are aware and awake in this moment, in the here and now.

I have found that meditation can make you sleepy if you close your eyes. For this reason I always keep my eyes open. When doing so it is important at first to fixate on a specific point. This allows you to turn off your thoughts and still be wide awake, fresh and at peace after meditation.


## For free or just for nothing

It was exasperating. I had received a call from a nice person who knew the details of my personal situation and knew that my increased health was due to my new lifestyle and diet. This meant always eating fresh, vitamin-rich food, basic food, etc., etc., etc.

We happily told each other what we were preparing for our next meals. He then told me innocently that he had two roulades wrapped in foil in his refrigerator that he was simply going to heat up. I knew he had not said this to annoy me, but it still made me sad.

I had talked myself hoarse several times over the years with friends and relatives, explaining how damaging reheated food is for our bodies. I became exhausted telling people how extremely harmful aluminium foil is for our food (particularly when it comes into direct contact with it), for our blood and finally for our brains.

Although I am the know-it-all in the family I did not say anything this time. I felt a certain resignation (or was it wisdom?).

As soon as anyone had any kind of ailment they all came straight to me expecting help. Everyone who knew me knew about the dangers of toxification. They all knew about the supposedly healthy lifestyles advertised in a way that was misleading and, yes, a lie. They all knew about the importance of a diet rich in vitamins and minerals without E numbers, artificial or chemical substances, sweeteners, glutamate and aluminium foil. And then something like this happens.


## Lavender alcohol and lavender oil

I have already spoken about making St John's wort oil. Lavender oil is made according to the same principle. Lavender alcohol which is rubbed into the solar plexus (the area under the breastbone and the upper stomach with the thymus gland in the centre) or used to massage the head and temples has a particularly calming effect. Hay flower oil, arnica oil and other helpful herbal oils can also be made in the same way. These home-made oils should only ever be used externally. As already mentioned, they are very easy to make.
Take a clear glass bottle and fill half of it with lavender flowers. You can use freshly picked lavender or dried lavender that you can buy at a pharmacy. Fill the bottle up with clear, 40 percent alcohol and leave it for 6 weeks in a light, sunny place. Shake it thoroughly two to three times a week. After six weeks, strain it and decant it into small, dark bottles that can be sealed tightly.


## Dark field microscopy

In the spring I was given another pointer by a friend from Switzerland who had heard that I was collecting data and facts about Parkinson's disease to pass on to other Parkinson's sufferers at a later date.
He asked me if had heard about dark field microscopy. Yes, I had heard about it, but only in connection with cancer.
This friend knew an alternative practitioner who had opened a dark field microscopy centre and who was also able to recognise the disease patterns of Parkinson's disease, Alzheimer's disease and multiple sclerosis in the blood and use homeopathic methods to treat them. Of course I was curious to learn something new and to have a new

perspective of the severity of my disease and a new definition of it. By now I felt very well on some days but I still felt again and again that my disease was still affecting me.
To make a long story short, I made an appointment.
I was more than surprised.

A drop of blood was gently taken from my middle finger and placed between two glass sides, which were placed under the dark field microscope. This special microscope has a 1600x magnification. My little drop of blood was around $1cm^2$ in size.
The magnified image was displayed on a monitor. What I saw was a tiny section of around $1mm^2$, but magnified to fill the full monitor. Until then I had thought of the mountains or the ocean as nature's greatest wonder. I had to revise this opinion.
What I saw in my $1mm^2$ section of blood was breath-taking. Now it became clear to me that nature's greatest wonder is us. Everything that was going on in there was explained to me in detail. There were red and white blood cells swimming around. Some were active, some were empty shells because they had been hollowed out or attacked by viruses. Some of them had a drop of oxygen in the middle. And there were small gold clumps – mercury – or beautiful blue crystals – aluminium – and other crystals that stood out that were my acids.
Fungi were creating new threads to form new nests and store heavy metals and toxins in them.
I could not believe what I was seeing. This drop of blood was then analysed using radionics, a form of testing devised by Bruce Copen, to get a full picture of my blood.
Over the following days, the blood was analysed each day and the data was recorded.
Here it is worth mentioning that our blood lives for several days; my blood lived, reacted and tried to destroy bacteria and fungi for 11 days between the glass slides.
I was very impressed.
In this context, it is interesting that practitioners of conventional

medicine are convinced that our drops of blood are sterile and only live for one day. Strange… this property of blood was discovered by various scientists almost 200 years ago.

Professor Günther Enderlein spread the word in Germany about his discovery back in 1916. His first publications followed in 1925. In his works he refuted the teachings of Professor R. Virchow who maintained that blood was sterile.

My blood had now been analysed. Subsequently, a special course of homeopathic medication as part of a course of detoxification was created for me. I followed it diligently for the next 12 weeks. After all, I wanted to get rid of the annoying 'lodgers' that were making me ill. The crucial point here is that all of the viruses, bacteria and other things that cause illness are targeted and flushed out, and not, as is usually the case in conventional medicine, killed off with antibiotics. This is because, unfortunately, the chemical antibiotic treatments also kill useful viruses, bacteria and other things that we desperately need, such as those in the intestine. In all my homeopathic course of detoxification with various medications lasted over a year, until I was told that everything was normal and they could do nothing more for me.


**Daily routine during my course of detoxification (12 weeks)**

**6 a.m. get up**

Measure pH level =        week 1 daily: 5.9
                          week 2 daily: 6.2–6.5

1 hour of swimming
Shower with Fortakehl, Rebas or Alibicansan
alternately

Nasal rinse with basic salt
Drink 1 small glass of healing water from Lourdes
Use 1 small glass of healing water from Lourdes for head massage

Singing bowl therapy
1 glass of fresh sage tea
Meditation

### 9.30 a.m. breakfast

Porridge made of wild brown top millet, spelt flakes, wheat bran,
linseed, poppy seeds, coconut flakes, whey and fresh mixed fruit, e.g.
banana, pineapple, papaya, apricot, mango, pomegranate, persimmon,
red grapes, passion fruit, various nuts, etc. with Greek yoghurt (6–
10% fat, made of sheep's milk if possible), honey and pollen and a
glass of freshly squeezed orange and grapefruit juice

Every 30 minutes alternately:
Rizol, Osiba, wild garlic or coriander, chlorella, rye

### 1 p.m. lunch

Bread, raw vegetables, e.g. carrots, lettuce, tomatoes, radishes,
olives, no processed meat products – instead vegetarian spread, basil
and garlic pesto, etc.
1 tsp Wurzelkraft and/or home-made spread, e.g. with avocado,
tapenade (olive spread)
7 x 7 herbal tea and different kinds of good quality water

### 3 p.m. coffee break

1 cup of coffee and a glass of water – not ideal but I did not want to cut
out every little pleasure; a biscuit or some bread and jam

Then alternately:
Wild garlic or coriander mother tincture
Rye , Osiba, chlorella, Rizol
1 small glass of mineral water followed by meditation
2x per week: one hour of yoga
1x per week: alkaline bath after Baunscheidt therapy (This therapy
uses a small hand-held roller with little wheels covered in tiny

needles. You use it to piece the skin to get the maximum effect of the bath. Ideally it should be used until tiny drops of blood appear.)

Every other week an alkaline enema

### 8 p.m. dinner
With cooked vegetables, potatoes, carrots, ginger, garlic, onions, artichokes, tomatoes, peppers, cabbages, fennel, possibly some couscous, red rice, pasta, etc.
Possibly some organic fish or a very small amount of organic poultry: maximum 1 or 2 times per week

### 11 p.m. go to bed
Before bed: nasal rinse with alkaline bath
Liver massage with St John's wort oil/lavender
oil, Mucedokehl, Froximun (clinoptilolite)

### ... and during the entire course
No alcohol, instead 7 x 7 tee or another alkaline tea, healing water with a few drops of $H_2O_2$

If feeling hungry: organic apple chips, fruit, etc.
I found a few articles about dark field microscopy online. They sounded like crime novels.
On the subject of crime novels, the story of another dark field microscopy researcher, Dr Wilhelm von Brehmer, reads like a gruesome thriller.[40] Dr von Brehmer was head of the pathological microbiology laboratories in Berlin in 1923.
Here he discovered the significance of the pH level in bodily fluids. His first publications on the subject appeared in 1928 and 1931. In 1932, he published his thesis entitled 'Krebs – eine Erregerkrankheit' (cancer – a disease caused by pathogens). This work was presented in a special edition of the magazine *Medizinische Welt* in 1934 and every point was backed up by Professor V. Schilling, the head and

director of the university hospital in Berlin-Moabit.
Due to his popularity Dr von Brehmer was invited to join the Nazi party, which he declined to do. After this his work was described as unscientific and fantastical. Dr von Brehmer was banned from publishing anything. He subsequently set up the Paracelsus Institute in Nuremberg which, due to its successes in healing, was shut down in 1937 at Hitler's demand. However, influential figures from industry, such as, Robert Bosch and Hugo Stinnes, continued to support his work.

## Other treatments – dark field microscopy II

After eight more weeks of the course of treatment a new image was taken of my blood using dark field microscopy.
There were positive tendencies. The values for trichomonads, heavy metals and camouflaged candida (C-candida, see below), to name just a few, were much better than they were the first time. Suddenly there were empty spaces visible in the blood. On the basis of her experience the alternative practitioner suspected that I had a dead tooth that had had root canal treatment, which I confirmed.
Who likes the idea of a corpse in their dining room?
Now the negative effect that root canal treatments have on our blood and our bodies as a whole was made clear to me, along with the natural methods of dealing with them through a combined treatment carried out by a dentist and a foot reflexology therapist. This is because each tooth stands for a particular organ in the body that can be influenced by the reflex zones in the feet.

In this context, another article that I read a while ago comes to mind. It was about root canal treatment.[41] It explained how teeth causing problems that had had root canal treatment could be successfully injected with procaine by a dentist who specialises in natural medicine. It may be an alternative to root canal treatment.

The book *Candidalismus?!* (candidalism) by Sabine and Ekkehard Scheller helped me begin to understand the connections within the body.[42] It is written is a very clear, descriptive and understandable way.
With a great deal of personal commitment, the alternative practitioner Ekkehard Scheller has re-established dark field microscopy as a technology in Germany and Switzerland. He once said at a health conference, 'Disease is a healthy way to discover ourselves.'

We should be thankful for these signals that our body is sending us, as a disease or symptom is a crucial indicator that we must change something in our bodies.
Using dark field microscopy, in addition to the number of red and white blood cells, we can see viruses, leeches, fungi and other bad things, as well as what are known as symbionts. These are tiny white dots that can only be seen using dark field microscopy and whizz around the screen. These symbionts (symbiosis = balance) create the balance between health and disease throughout our lives. They are made of protein and are the foundation of all living things. Each symbiont has a storage capacity equal to two human brains.

The individual character of the symbionts shapes the individual being according to God's plan.[43] This is a quote from Ekkehard Scheller.
We are the ecosystem in which all of this happens! We can think of blood as a kind of primordial soup. The symbionts often continue to live in the blood for several weeks after death. In dark field microscopy it is the blood that provides the information. The blood terrain is determined by our red and white blood cells and oxygen, but also by pollutants such as acids, heavy metals, bacteria, viruses and fungi. Borellia, for example, are often responsible for depression. They usually cannot be seen in the cells. In the blood we often find what are known as C-tricho-monads or C-candida, which were discovered by Ekkhard Scheller.[44]

According to Ekkehard Scheller, the C stands for camouflage, as these are camouflaged form of pathogens and fungi. In healthy people they are normally found uncamouflaged in the intestine where they have an important function, but they have no place in our blood. However, as they have mutated through a porous intestinal wall they have become camouflaged and found their way into the blood, where they cause various diseases and weaken the immune system. There were also other tips in the book by Sabine and Ekkehard Scheller that led me to new ideas. For example, it describes the Rechtsregulat products made by the company Dr. Niedermaier Pharma and their fascinating potential to reorganise, repair and have restorative effects on the body (see the following passage).


## Rechtsregulat

Fermentation helps to activate what are known as unlocked enzymes in our bodies. Rechtsregulat is a regulator that helps this process. In nature, celeriac, lemons, shoots, walnuts, onions and artichokes, among other things, also act as regulators.

At the time of birth and during breastfeeding everyone gets a large supply of enzymes. This supply of enzymes should be maintained. Unfortunately, however, poor nutrition, a lack of exercise, stress, electro smog, chemical medications and many other factors cause these enzymes to disappear. Global studies suggest that over 80 percent of the population suffers from a lack of vital substances and enzymes.[45] When early harvests and long storage times for unripe fruit and vegetables cause a loss of vital enzymes, taking Rechtsregulat early and regularly restores our internal balance. Rechtsregulat contains symbionts (see part I, Dark field microscopy II) that are very similar to those found in the human body. This means that they also have direct access to the immune system. Rechtsregulat energises each individual cell and brings up energy levels to the original level required for the metabolism, to remove heavy metals in the autoimmune system and in the hormone system for an alkaline lifestyle. It can be ingested or absorbed through the skin.

I have come to the conclusion that Rechtsregulat products are especially important for Parkinson's patients. They are able to counteract a lack of vitamins and minerals, have a noticeable effect on build-ups of waste and pesticides that poison the body and paralyse the nervous system, and help to promote detoxification.[46] Rechtsregulat was a key part of my later courses of therapy (see part II, 5, Blood health; 6, Intestinal health; 24, Rechtsregulat).

## A visit to the doctor

I had another routine visit to the doctor. I felt good. The doctor greeted me cheerfully saying, 'Wow, you look good! Are you still taking the pills I prescribed you?'

That got me thinking that what she might really have meant was 'How can you look so good taking *those* pills?'

Should I have told her that I had not been taking any psychotropic drugs for a month? Instead I told her that I wanted to stop taking the psychotropic drugs because I no longer thought they were necessary.

## Chronically ill patients

While watching television I discovered that due to health reforms statutory health insurance providers had been paying insurance contributions from citizens into a health fund since 2008.

This fund is used to give each health insurance provider tax payers' money based largely on the number of chronically ill patients that they have. They are given additional funding by the state (i.e. the tax payer) for each person who is proven to be chronically ill.

This is a major disadvantage for patients, as it means that chronically ill patients like me can no longer change health insurance providers. As a chronically ill patient, no private health insurance providers would take me after finding out from my statutory health insurance provider that I had Parkinson's disease and was taking medications that included antidepressants which contained the notorious active ingredient fluoxetine (see Side Effects: Death[47]).


## Therapy devices

When visiting a Swiss friend of mine I was introduced to how to use the PowerTube and the QuickZap from Martin Frischknecht.
As I had discovered Dr Clark's direct current zapper[48] in 2006, I was not surprised to hear about this potential therapy. However, these devices that I was shown used alternating current impulses in the overtone scales. They were developed by Martin Frischknecht from Switzerland as TENS devices.[49] After using the PowerTube for several weeks I felt good operating it. I used it mainly to stimulate my large intestine, liver and pancreas to support the process of purging heavy metals, leeches, worms and the like from my body that was being carried out by the homeopathic medicines.

They can be used for a whole range of diseases and symptoms – from Alzheimer's disease to blood disease, fibromyalgia, Parkinson's disease, and inflammation of the teeth and jaw – and I have made a list of examples with details of suggested treatment (see references: *Gesundheit als Chance*[50]).
*A note from other users:* Smokers and/or those with severe overacidification have sometimes experienced temporary worsening of symptoms.


## Garlic cure

Someone suggested a garlic cure to purify and thin my blood. Blood has to supply the nerves with oxygen and needs to make it into the tiniest branches in the brain. The treatment cleans the veins from the inside and removes plaques without leaving a trace. Blood pressure is restored to normal. It is an all-in-one package for your health. The treatment is especially useful where there is damage, such as that caused by Parkinson's disease.

In 1971, a Unesco team found a recipe for a garlic cure written on clay tablets in a ruined monastery in Tibet. The team translated the recipe into many different languages.

A garlic cure frees the body of all build-ups of fat and lime scale. It improves the metabolism and preserves the elasticity of the blood vessels. It also helps prevent heart attacks (caused by blockages in arteries), sclerosis, stenocardia, angina, tinnitus, strokes and cancer. Vision is also improved.

I strongly recommend this treatment to everyone, especially those suffering from Parkinson's and Alzheimer's disease and people who have suffered a stroke. The effect on blood flow in the brain, the arteries of which are split into many fine branches, was noticeable after just a few weeks in my case.

Preparation:
Peel 250g of fresh garlic. Crush it and put it into 200g of 90% alcohol (available from pharmacies). Put the mixture into a sealed jar and store in a cool place for 10 days. Then filter the mixture through a cloth, making sure the garlic is thoroughly squeezed out. After three days you can begin treatment.

Use:
Put the drops into a glass with 50ml of room-temperature milk (soy, oat, spelt or coconut milk). I alternate between oat, spelt and/or almond milk, which cause less of a garlicy smell and aftertaste.

Dosage:
Take with meals

|        | Breakfast | Lunch | Dinner |
|--------|-----------|-------|--------|
| Day 1  | 1 drop    | 2 drops  | 3 drops  |
| Day 2  | 4 drops   | 5 drops  | 6 drops  |
| Day 3  | 7 drops   | 8 drops  | 9 drops  |
| Day 4  | 10 drops  | 11 drops | 12 drops |
| Day 5  | 13 drops  | 14 drops | 15 drops |
| Day 6  | 15 drops  | 14 drops | 13 drops |
| Day 7  | 12 drops  | 11 drops | 10 drops |
| Day 8  | 9 drops   | 8 drops  | 7 drops  |
| Day 9  | 6 drops   | 5 drops  | 4 drops  |
| Day 10 | 3 drops   | 2 drops  | 1 drops  |

From day 11 onwards, take 25 drops in 50ml of milk three times a day with meals until all of the mixture has been used.
It is recommended that this treatment is carried out twice a year.

## Follow up examination and treatment – dark field microscopy III

My blood was examined again using dark field microscopy. Another 12 weeks had gone by. Everyone was very pleased. My alternative practitioner said that I now needed to do the rest. She wanted to encourage me considering that I had been following the course of treatment very exactly and sticking closely to the time schedule for months. Every 20 to 30 minutes I had taken a specific preparation without complaining. I could see the results and it had been worth it. Even my Parkinson's factor had improved.
Now my metabolism had to start doing its job again. In order for this to happen I was supposed to inject myself in the thigh with

three different ampoules for ten weeks. Now I felt a little differently. The pharmacy in Switzerland had sent everything. Now I had to learn how to prepare and carry out an injection. Just opening the ampoule is difficult enough for a layperson.
I looked for help and found a very helpful doctor who I explained my problem to. The packaging explained that this injection needed to be administered subcutaneously (under the skin). She showed me how to inject three ampoules one after the other into a fold of skin by myself. It was a new experience but it is possible to get used to anything.
It is difficult to describe the effects I experienced in the final few weeks. Every day was different. Sometimes I still experienced severe problems. Walking was difficult. Thinking required a great deal of effort. Dizziness and slowness were a problem on some days. However, as my wellbeing went from one extreme to the other, I feel that the worsening symptoms had healing effects. Writing, researching for and thinking about this book gave me a great deal of strength and confidence in myself.

Then suddenly there was a crisis.
In the fourth week of my course of injections my body rebelled. Around five hours after the injections I felt incredibly sick. Large amounts of liquid collected in my mouth to such an extent that I could not spit them out quickly enough. All of my abdominal organs rebelled, my liver swelled, my spleen hurt and my kidneys were sounding the alarm.
I told the alternative practitioner about this. She immediately sent me globules of a strength that I did not believe would do anything, C 1000.
However, I knew that the C 200 and C 1000 strengths were used very often by Dr Samuel Hahnemann, the founder of homeopathic medicine. The first time I took them I felt almost exactly the same as I had after the injections. However, after two days the globules made the situation more and more bearable, allowing me to continue the course of injections.

I experienced some rather interesting reactions. For example, sometimes I felt as though sand was running over my head, as though the meridian points on the back of my head were pulsing, or as if someone was pulling a cloth or a woolly hat over my head. It was very strange! However, as it did not hurt it was bearable, and I trusted in my treatment and its healing.

As I know that we are guided, I tried to learn from my disease. Why had I developed this disease that had ruined me financially and physically six years ago? Where did the feeling that I had had for the past year that I would be able to become healthy again, or at least healthy enough that I could start taking part in everyday activities again, come from?
My daily meditation helped me to have patience and to gratefully accept the small steps towards healing that I had been given from the universe of my creator. After all, disease is a spiritual act.
I felt as though I could set something in motion. Not in my old profession, but there were people who might need me and who I might be able to help. I had learnt, used and experienced so much over the past few years that it could be helpful for others to speak about their disease with me.
To learn and share with others how to accept and understand disease, however bad it may be. Why do I feel like this and how am I? Our diseases are a reflection of our lives. When we have finally understood this it is unfortunately often too late for a quick solution. I often had the painful experience that others looking for help talked a great deal and grasped at sometimes rather questionable methods that were supposed to help but were not prepared to actively contribute to helping, to accept the disease and to fight against it by changing their diet and giving up cigarettes, alcohol and the other dangerous excesses found in our society.

## A medal

As my wife and I were discussing  pharmaceuticals again and the
studies on them by some professors and other hired mouthpieces
who have been bought by the pharmaceutical industry she said, 'You
known, the physiotherapist that advised you not to take chemical
medications years ago really deserves a medal!'
I can still remember the situation very clearly but unfortunately I
cannot mention this caring and brave woman's name as I do not wish
to cause her any difficulties. Nevertheless, I will be eternally grateful
to her.
At the time she asked me during a treatment which medications I had
to take. I told her the names. There were many, including fluoxetine,
which is now rather infamous but was almost unknown then. I could
not see the therapist as I was lying on my stomach but I felt her
hesitate. Very quietly and in a very sad voice she said, 'I'm not allowed
to say what I'm about to say as it would cost me my job here. But last
week my mother died from taking these medications.'

*That was the crucial turning point in my life.*


## A medical insider speaks out

This turning point became even clearer when, several days later, I
was given a book recommendation and ordered the recommended
book myself. Somehow it reminded me of my marathon of reviews
and discussions with experts. The book was *Ein medizinischer Insider
packt aus*[51] (a medical insider speaks out) by Professor Peter Yoda.
Yoda is the pseudonym of a German university professor who used to
be the head of a German university hospital and was a long-term
member of a scientific association. The book was published as a novel,
probably to cover the author's tracks. It is written very clearly, making
it easy to understand for laypeople.

Yoda describes a transformation which is as drastic as St Paul's on the road to Damascus. When the author, professor at a university and a doctor of conventional medicine, gets cancer himself, he and his wife begin to have serious doubts about current common methods of treatment. He looks for help and advice at a special scientific association that explains to him the developments of chemotherapy and the medications involved, whether it is used for cancer, AIDS or everyday diseases.

Yoda receives information about how politicians, the pharmaceutical industry and doctors scare the public so that we are prepared to tolerate and pay for these pointless toxins that make us ill.

The book explains what the galas for cancer charities are really about and why this fear that it could affect us or our children is deliberately created. But as long as more and more people can profit more and more from cancer and cancer treatment it will continue to be this way.

In Professor Yoda's book we meet renowned scientists from countries such as Russia, China and the USA who are now taking different approaches, with considerable success. However, according to the author these people and scientists live in fear of having a sudden 'accident' if their research is ever published because it would be inconvenient for certain politicians and for the pharmaceutical industry!

For me the most important part of the book is where it says that no one in this world is interested in making sick people healthy again unless the healing process generates many costs.[52]

But it does not have to be like this. The book discusses the possibilities of cell and organ regeneration. It also cautiously tells the reader about spiritual guidance and the powers of self-healing that are in all of us.

Several non-fiction books by various authors from the same publisher as listed in the appendix. This book is incredibly important for anyone who has not considered the lies and false information spread by the pharmaceutical industry until now.

## Parkinson's clinic

One weekend I had the opportunity fulfil a promise that I had made some time ago to visit and exchange ideas with someone. An acquaintance of mine who was also suffering from Parkinson's disease was spending some time at a Parkinson's clinic.

As in the meantime my condition had started worsening again, it was not easy for me to see and speak to all of these people, some of whom were in wheelchairs, who needed so much help.

The thought went through my head that, according to the calculations of my doctors from 2003 and 2004, I should also have been sitting in a wheelchair. I was thankful for my fate and the associated 'coincidences' and full of empathy for the patients in the clinic.

My acquaintance showed me and my wife around the clinic. His wife had also come to visit and had baked a cake. We took our time and had a long discussion. In the generous, light and friendly atmosphere, which made the place seem pleasant from the moment you entered, there was hardly a trace of the daily routine of therapy.

In the clinic's library I searched without success for literature on how natural therapies can be used to treat Parkinson's disease or at least as a complementary therapy. I found nothing. Instead I found only brochures from various doctors about which drugs should be taken when, and which medications could be used to supress side effects.

The icing on the cake came from our acquaintance when he told us about his latest medications that the doctor had made extra attractive by telling him that these brand new capsules were not available anywhere else. 'Not even the pharmacy has them! They're the latest and best thing for Parkinson's disease right now.'

There were various printed copies of ARD reports from World Parkinson's Day 2009 lying around. They did not give any hope either. They also said that Parkinson's disease could not be cured. Pesticides and medications were acknowledged as possible causes, in addition to accidents and allergies. At least there were no more citations of the story about the boxer Muhammed Ali who had one too many knocks on the head that I had been told years before. One

article commented that the cause was currently unknown. Other
brochures once again sang the praises of the newest procedures in
nuclear medicine, such as DaTSCAN or PET. These had been around
for years when people had radioactive contrast substances injected
into them, which was essentially radioactive pollution of the body.
What I do not understand in all of this is why medical staff in Germany
do not have any guidelines for themselves during and after the
treatment, as is the case for all staff at the university hospital in Vienna
who deal with these materials. When will conventional medicine
understand that Parkinson's disease is *not* a causative disorder of the
brain but that the sick brain is only a symptom of the disease? When I
say 'sick brain', I mean the symptoms that cause the lack of dopamine
in the substantia nigra. For doctors the cause is Parkinson's disease.
However, in my opinion and according to my own experience, it is just a
symptom, as Parkinson's disease is caused by toxification of the body
due to food, medications, the environment and other factors.
The liver is affected first, then the blood and then the brain, which
ultimately stops producing dopamine. This leads to the familiar loss of
function in the brain, the nerves and the muscles. The doctor simply
prescribes the Parkinson's sufferer dopamine replacements and
antidepressants because he does not know about or accept the disease
of the organs, for whatever reason.
Of course the treatments and methods used at the Parkinson's clinic,
be they creative therapies, speech therapy or physiotherapy, are very
important and very helpful for the patients. Older people and those
who are sick need to drink a lot, that is true, but is it not important
that they are drinking the right things?
It is generous to have unlimited bottled mineral water available, but
why do people give patients carbonated water? The information that
this water is not recommended for sick people (or for those who
consider themselves still healthy) should have got around in medical
circles by now. Carbon dioxide is an acid that influences the acidity
levels in the body. Of course, the pharmacists have pills and powder to
treat overacidity. How clever!

My acquaintance told me about a big survey being carried out by a
neurology clinic with an interdisciplinary centre for palliative medicine.
I was given a copy of the survey and was appalled. This may have
initially been due to the words used. In the survey, palliative medicine
was seen as the final stage for Parkinson's patients. And it really is
final, as is clear in from the following definition found in the
Psychrembel medical dictionary (translated from the original German):
'Palliative medicine (lat. palliare, to cover with a coat): active, holistic
treatment of a progredient, very advanced disease that cannot be
cured; the alleviation of pain, other complaints and psychological,
social and spiritual problems have the highest priority in palliative
medicine. The goal is to maintain the best possible quality of life
through the best possible pain therapy and symptom control. The
autonomy of the patient should be respected; relatives' needs should
be considered. Open, sympathetic communication between the patient,
relatives and specialists is required. The dying process is neither
actively accelerated nor artificially slowed down. See hospice, assisted
dying.'[53]
Luckily most patients do not know what the term palliative medicine
means.

Back to the survey from the Parkinson's clinic mentioned above. After
the initial questions about gender, age and family situation were
questions about medication, such as bromocriptine, Seroxat, Zoloft, and
zolpidem. After asking about symptoms and possible questions
regarding diagnosis, questions about the Parkinson's sufferer's
financial situation were then unexpectedly included. Does that really
have a place in a medical survey? However, what I considered the
most outrageous thing was yet to come. The questionnaire gave
patients two possibilities for 'participation'. Here are the translations
of the direct quotes: 'I would like to take part in studies in which
medications are trialled as treatment' and 'I would be willing to
donate my brain to science for the disease to be researched after my
death.'

For me personally the only question that I had was what the clinic
would pay me to act as a guinea pig for medications that had not been
approved or to carry out investigations after my death. That would at
least be an opportunity to do something good with the pharmaceutical
industry's money.
Of course there was the option of answering no to both questions.


## Atlas therapy

After a long period of peace and quiet I once again had had bad pain
in my lower back for two days and could feel how my nerves were
on edge and suffering from it.
The previous night I had had a dream that took me back 30 years into
the past. Back then I had suffered terrible stress that came with bad
pain in my lower back and the surrounding muscles. I was given many
injections for it.
Today I finally know what had happened to me then.
In 2007, I had had atlas correction carried out. The therapist had
explained to me that it would be as if I was experiencing my whole,
partly painful life in reverse but speeded up, as if someone had
pressed a rewind button. It was calculated that I would need around
one month of therapy per year of my life.
This all became clear to me. As the body and mind do not forget, I
was transported back to 30 years before over the course of these
weeks. This realisation encouraged me as it meant that I would
soon have overcome this episode.
My current therapy was a massage with warming muscle oil and a
wool blanket wrap; otherwise the important thing was movement,
movement, movement. In the afternoons I would do more yoga and
of course an energy transfer as part of my daily meditation.

Things would be better from now on! I felt good again.

## Dr Shioya's universal therapy

Dr Nobuo Shioya (born 1902) is considered a pioneer in holistic methods of achieving a 'fountain of youth' effect with universal energy.[54] He is now 107 years old and still plays golf, and has been a doctor and teacher of Japanese wisdom for decades. Since his youth he has worked with various breathing and meditation techniques to speed up the powers of healing within us (and therefore within the universe, as he believes we are part of the universe) and maintain them throughout our lifetimes.

According to the principle of attraction we can affect our health through positive imagination, simply through our thoughts. According to Dr Shioya, in combination with a good breathing technique, similar to those used in yoga exercises but more intense and direct, we can achieve amazing results. His method is very easy to apply for anyone who is open to this approach.

The most important rules are simple:
Think positively about everything.
Never forget to give thanks.
Do not complain.

Dr Shioya offers a therapy without any form of medication that 'only' uses the power of the mind. It is a therapy that anyone can apply for themselves.

As I had been learning how to work with universal energy and elementary meditation since 2007, I found these suggestions and possibilities very interesting. I am sure I would not have got this book to read if I had not actually needed it.
In his book Nobuo Shioya describes the universal power. He describes this endless power of the universe that created the countless planets in space, for example.
'Where does this universal power come from then?' most people ask.

Indeed, where does this power come from that is so
incomprehensibly large and tremendous? It is simply there. Just like
our good, caring thoughts that can cause a 'miracle', that let our
thoughts and wishes come true; through the law of attraction.
Over 2000 years ago, Matthew wrote, 'If you believe, you will receive
whatever you ask for in prayer' (Matthew 21:22). Mark reported the
words of Christ, 'When you pray and ask for something, believe that
you have received it, and you will be given whatever you ask for'
(Mark 11:24).
These verses correspond to my new experiences in life. Of course it is
very difficult to always control your thoughts in medication and in
prayer. It requires practice and concentration. But it is certainly
always worth a try.

So stick with it and practice! I have experienced myself that it works
when the need is greatest because then there is no room for any
other thoughts. The second step is trust. If I only trust strongly
enough that my request will be fulfilled then it has already happened,
exactly as it is described in the verses above. It is not easy to
understand but please do not doubt it!


## The healing arts of tomorrow

I was told about a book by Erika Herbst and her self-help group,
Mündiger Bürger e.V., called *Die Lösung des Krebsproblems – Die
Heilkunst von Morgen*[55] (solving the cancer problem – the healing arts
of tomorrow). Ms Herbst sent me a copy of the book, as it can only be
order through the self-help group. The courage and commitment with
which this woman investigates diseases and their causes is
astounding. It is truly impressive.
I will provide a summary of her contribution to the search for the
cause of and treatment for Parkinson's disease here.
According to Erika Herbst, the causes of Parkinson's disease are
largely to do with geopathical factors. Based on her experience,

however, it has less to do with water veins and earth grids and more to do with earth grid crossings that are near to where the patient sleeps.
In these places the electrical burden is extremely high. This is increased by the alternating magnetic field in electrical wires in the walls and through the position of plug sockets. Ms Herbst also describes the extremely negative, toxic effect of medications, genetic disposition, vaccinations, dental metal, metabolic toxins, environmental toxins, and other potential factors of disease. Overacidification is also a key focus of her research into causes. According to patient reports and readers' letters in her book, taking the product Kanne Brottrunk every day and regularly eating fermented grain from the brand Demeter led to significant improvement of symptoms. Especially in the early stages of disease this meant that the dosages of Parkinson's medication could be kept to a minimum.

Lymph drainage and foot reflexology, two things I have already discussed above, were also mentioned by Ms Herbst.
There are many other suggestions in Erika Herbst's book. Dr Hans Selzer believes that Parkinson's diseases is a disease of the lymph system. In a book by Stefanie Achleitner called *Schüttellähmung und Multiple Sklerose* (the shaking palsy and multiple sclerosis), the author suggests a tried and tested combination of seven homeopathic methods that reduce inflammation and five methods that regulate lymphatism. She also discusses urine therapy.
As a whole, Erika Herbst's book offers a collection of information about the potential of natural treatment and healing for cancer and many other diseases, as well as detailed research into causes based on experience and observation. It is a fantastic book, full of love, commitment and expertise, with all the information in one place and unparalleled in clarity!
Here is a translation of a quote from the book: 'If, however, you continue to take your poisonous brain medication, you do not need to

bother with the "healing arts of tomorrow", because if you want to put out the fire of disease you must not relight the fire every day. Modern medicine tries to kill diseases with poisons, which ends up poisoning the whole person. The "healing powers of tomorrow", on the other hand, heal the affected organs. And they do not need any kind of poison.'[56]

Finally, I would like to pass on a warning from the book: the Parkinson's medication Tasmar from LaRoche has already caused at least three deaths.[57]

# 2010–The right decision – recovery is noticeable

## Healing

In the first half of January I once again experienced difficulties walking, thinking and moving in general.

It was nothing compared to how I had felt five years ago, but it was not how I had felt over the last three months. I was simply a bit awkward, dazed or unsure. My thinking and reactions had become slower again. When the telephone rang I became anxious. I lost concentration very quickly. My wife confirmed that I was once again veering to the right when I walked. I just wanted to be left in peace. One afternoon after a two-hour nap, during which I slept deeply, I felt much better. However, over the past two nights I had experienced some very strange things. Each night between 3 and 4 a.m. I suddenly sneezed, spluttered and snorted. My nose ran and ran. Inside my head I could feel how the phlegm in my sinuses ran into my throat and oesophagus. It was very unpleasant but it did not hurt.

This lasted almost two days and prevented me from falling back asleep. However, I did not have any symptoms of a cold. What was it? It was the effects of a little indulgence over the holidays.

Over the past month I had allowed myself the occasional glass of wine, a cup of coffee or something sweet – more often than normal. The two kilogrammes of weight I had put on spoke for themselves. It is what happens over the holidays. When I had been invited to friends' houses I had eaten some sausages or a little meat. I did not want to make a fuss. This was really just proof that in Parkinson's patients the toxins and acids that are contained in these treats accumulate inside the head. This happened despite my weekly alkaline baths.

I decided to use my alkaline baths and alkaline socks multiple times over the next few days to detoxify. A few days of eating half as much as normal would do the rest to bring me back into my old shape. For several weeks, my nose ran for around an hour every morning, even though I did not have a cold. It just did. After a few more weeks I had the impression that I could smell better again. I had hoped for that. I had trusted that it would happen. I believed very strongly in it.

Healing comes from God; it is a holy action, and the two words 'healing' and 'holy' share the same roots.


## Brain pacemaker

The December 2009 issue of *Apotheken Umschau* magazine claimed that after taking medication with massive side effects for six to eight years, Parkinson's patients could still play tennis or do similar activities. Exceptions were possible.[58]
However, many cases prove that this is usually not possible. The magazine claimed that patients first experienced difficulties with writing after ten years. Yet studies have shown that most Parkinson's patients are no longer able to write legibly after just three to five years.
I believe that here, once again, people are being told the classic misconception that the cause of Parkinson's disease lies in the brain. My experiences have shown something quite different.
The magazine described how neurons in the midbrain that produce the messenger substance dopamine, which in turn controls the muscles, for example, die off. While this is a rather simplified description, it is absolutely correct. Based on my experience, I believe that this is just a symptom of Parkinson's disease and not the cause.
Of course, the side effects of Parkinson's medication, anti-depressants and other drugs and their effects on our organs were not mentioned. Now a chip was supposed to sort everything out.
I do not think that it is right to talk about deep brain simulation with a brain pacemaker in such a way as to make it seem harmless, or to actually talk about fantastic effects and improved quality of life when only the dosage of medication is focused on.
Of course it should be recognised if it improves aspects such as

pronunciation and brain activity considerably. However, it is important
to listen to the experts who say that long-term use of brain
pacemakers can disrupt thoughts and feelings and can cause
changes in the Patient's personality.


## Placebo

My great efforts to activate my own powers of self-healing and, on
the side, to look out for natural treatments and therapies and use
them if possible were met with a total lack of understanding by
doctors, and they responded simply by shaking their heads. They
were interested, as by now my very good general condition spoke
volumes, but they could not deal with it. They came up with terms
like 'placebo effect' and 'spontaneous healing'.
Placebo effects are laughed at by most doctors. In their eyes they
are a delusion that goes hand in hand with trivialising the severity of
a condition.
According to my experience the placebo effect (Lat.: placebo = I will
please) is something else. Meister Eckehart, a German 13th century
mystic, said, 'The ideas of the soul have a stronger effect on the body
than a doctor and his medications!' The placebo effect changes
something in the brain if I am convinced of it. This is also the
common view held by medical experts. However, it also means that
the psychological processes (the belief in healing) have their own
'biology' and can therefore bring about healing with the placebo. This
can also be called self-healing.

At the same time when several placebo medications did so well in the
pharmaceutical industry's tests that the chemical medications with
their many side effects no longer seemed necessary, a new term was
coined: the nocebo effect. As the December 2009 issue of the
magazine *Welt der Wunder* explains, the term nocebo refers to a self-
fulfilling negative prophecy.[59] This means that, just as with a placebo a
person's thoughts can make them healthy, negative thoughts

(Lat.: nocebo = I will harm) can make them ill.
This applies to all Parkinson's patients.

Studies by the cell biologist and nocebo researcher Bruce Lipton show
that an astonishing 70 percent of people's thoughts are negative.
According to Lipton, the effect of these negative influences has
catastrophic consequences for the body's biochemical functions. The
nocebo effect can cause damage throughout the entire body![60]
So when someone says, 'You have Parkinson's; it's an incurable disease,' this
surely has a nocebo effect. The patient is then probably no longer able to
believe in being healed. In some Parkinson's clinics and from some doctors,
patients have to hear such statements repeatedly – until they have to believe
them.
We now know that the official warnings on cigarette packets –
'Smoking kills' – can also produce a nocebo effect.[61] This increases
the risk of cancer.

The conclusion is that the nocebo effect makes millions for the
pharmaceutical industry every year.
Jerome Groopmann is an immunologist who teaches at Harvard
Medical School. His research clearly backs up his philosophy that the
most important tool for healing is the power of our brain – it is the
best pharmacy in the world.[62]
All evidence suggests that our brain is able to produce highly
effective substances that are light-years ahead of any
pharmaceutical preparations.
Most experts in conventional medicine see thoughts and feelings as
something of secondary importance. They are in the brain but are a
mixture of biochemical processes and electrical circuits that change
and develop and change us – positively with the placebo effect or
negatively with the nocebo effect.
We are simply what we believe. Given this choice, I of course believe
strongly in becoming healthy again!

There are well-known studies that were carried out on medical students and other people that tested whether participants thought red or blue placebo pills would have a stronger effect on healing. They always thought that the red pills had a warming, pleasant and stimulating effect, while the blue pulls had a calming, cooling and balancing effect.
It was therefore clearly the colour that influenced the psyche. For this reason, the people who design medications make sure that the colour of the medication corresponds exactly to its intended effects.
Scientific studies have shown that the placebo effect works incredibly well even in surgery. In an experiment carried out in the USA some patients had standard surgery for arthritis in the knee. Another group with the same number of patients with the same condition received and incision with visible sutures that simply simulated the surgery. In follow-up examinations two years later, 90 percent of both patient groups were happy with the results of the surgery. The number of patients who no longer had any symptoms was actually larger in the group with the fake surgery.[63]
Another study went even further.
Parkinson's patients had surgery where the top of the skull underwent minor drilling. After the surgery, the patients were told that live cells had been inserted. Just the idea of having received these live cells led to considerable improvement in their overall condition.[64] These studies also show that placebos can have a significant positive influence on serotonin metabolism in patients with depression. The effect on hormone metabolism was also shown as the immune defences were improved.

From my own experience, I know that I can stimulate my body and mind so strongly through meditation, as well as life-affirming suggestions and affirmations, that my body's defences are activated. No pills or operations are necessary. Everyone can do this with the power of their own thoughts. These exercises are easy to learn.
It is a wonderful experience to discover for yourself what you can

achieve. Even health is attainable if you wish for it from the bottom
of your heart and firmly believe in healing.
But think careful about what you wish for!
Consider it clearly before you formulate your wishes, as once you have
wished for something you cannot change it so easily. You can repeat your
wishes regularly, ideally during mediation or directly afterwards. This may
also enable you to imagine a clear picture of how your condition and the
desired process will look. These wishes, formed in peace, with balance and
with love, stimulate our natural powers of self-healing with which we can
overcome disease. We can all do it. I have experienced it myself but I have
also received many crucial pointers from therapists that have led me to the
next stage of my healing, enabling me to formulate my wishes more clearly.

We have been provided for; we must simply learn to accept it. Let us
finally activate our body's own 'pharmacies' to heal ourselves!
Paracelsus, the great Renaissance physician, formulated the first ideas
for holistic medicine in which powers of self-healing were highly
important. In his writings he says:

> *The mind is the master,*
> *the imagination is its tool*
> *and the body is the malleable*
> *material. Diseases of the body*
> *can be healed with the help of*
> *medication or through the*
> *power of the mind*
> *that works through the soul!*

Today we call this mind control.
So let us trust in the possibilities of the placebo within us that we can set free
with the powers of our thoughts. Our subconscious needs positive images.
However, the main thing is that we become healthy again and regain our zest
for life. And the doctors can laugh about what they think of as esoteric
rubbish...

## What if?

One of the most important things I realised during this year was that if, after my desperate please to God in 2006, I had immediately become healthy again, that would have been a miracle. However, my current point of view shows me that it is better when miracles take a little longer.
It was only in this way that I could slowly learn to change my life and my lifestyle. If I had been miraculously healed I would very probably have quickly slipped back into my old lifestyle that damaged my health and made me ill.
But this way?
I feel cared for, I feel loved, I feel guided, and all of this makes me feel safe. I am no longer afraid. My health improves every day. I no longer want to and will not change anything about my new positive lifestyle. I am accepted as I am, in the love and warmth of the endless light of my creator.


## Dark field microscopy follow-up (I)

It was finally time – spring was here. I could go back to Switzerland for dark field microscopy. Over the winter months I had sent my blood to Switzerland by post, sealed between two glass slides.
This time we took a good friend with us who wanted to find out about the possibilities of diagnosis using dark field microscopy for herself. She was convinced and started taking the tried-and-tested natural medications straight away.
My blood values, or more specifically my blood terrain, were now in a satisfactory condition after 10 months of treatment. However, as there is always room for improvement, I continued on a less intensive course of treatment that was set out for me. From now on Rechtsregulat was to be my main 'medication'.

I noticed that the familiar symptoms of Parkinson's were occurring less and less. In the notes in my diary I saw that in November and

December 2009 and in January 2010, I had still had one day each
month where it required great effort to coordinate my brain and my
movements. But it had only been one day each month.
What was that compared with the previous years!
And now?
During the year I began to also note the days when I felt particularly good,
as I wanted to think not only about the disease but also about my health. I
had to get used to this new way of thinking but to my delight I
discovered that the good days were becoming more and more
frequent. My head, my body, my consciousness and my new positive
aura were clear and were visible to others as a kind of external proof.
I felt comfortable in my own skin again.

My wife and I had another long discussion with the natural therapist.
During the examination it became clear that my spleen and pancreas
still had detectable physical problems. However, the cause was most
likely psychological. I would not be able to detoxify my body in the
best possible way and complete the process as long as I was still
holding on to my old problems and values. I had to recognise the
psychological causes with the help of the therapist in order to become
completely healthy again.


## Reconcile yourself with yourself first!

'Open your heart for love and for healing and then it can happen,'
my natural therapist said, 'Because: the fundamental principle of
medicine is love.' This simple statement by Paracelsus says it all.

My therapist showed me a whole new world of perspectives – those in a
visible, earthly world and those in a spiritual word. This helped me to
understand how we can transform old, burdensome values, integrate them
and heal them, and experience love, wisdom and light in this way.

During one therapy session I gained a better understanding of the two halves of my brain. First there is the male half of the brain with its mind that has been programmed in the past. This is the doer, the rational person who had always decided everything alone. This manifests itself in a life full of work in our careers and family lives, a life with pressing deadlines, stress and old disputes with our parents, partners or siblings. All of this causes constant restlessness in our minds, as all thoughts that permit or actually produce anger or other negative feelings come back to us like a boomerang. Whether or not these thoughts are justified is irrelevant. They are stored deep within us and make us ill mentally or even physically. The consequences are confused and disordered feelings.

These unresolved issues are like energy fields that have a negative effect inside us and prevent healing.

Suppressing them is not a solution; the problems will remain. Investigations show that they are responsible for up to 80 percent of current mental strain in sick people. These burdensome thoughts simple go round and round in our minds and we cannot find peace; they are just there. We cannot drown our problems. Problems are good swimmers!

Conversely, the female half of the brain is characterised by love, devotion and humility. It allows me to see my body as a temple in which I can see the source of love, which provides vitality for the soul. My brain was currently only using 20 percent of this ability.

I wanted to learn to steer my consciousness towards healing; to fully develop my five senses again as my creator intended.

Healing is integration and reconciliation with myself and my life so far. If I am able to do this, to really live out this belief, then I will also be able to reconcile myself with my future life and then my health can stabilise itself permanently.

To put it another way, as long as a person rejects themselves they hinder the process of becoming healthy again, the process of healing.

---

In relation to this, I heard about Dr Bösch, a brain researcher at the University of Zurich who later became head of the department of psychiatry at University Hospital Zurich. Dr Bösch gets to the heart of the issue in his lectures and books: disease helps. This means that disease helps us to find out that something needs to be changed.[65] With the knowledge of the possibilities in my brain and the significance of reconciliation I was now able to better understand the elements of holistic dark field microscopy: the body, mind and soul are one. I want to consciously work more on this in the future.

## What will health insurance cover?

It is our misfortune that we receive medications that are often laden with toxins from our health insurance providers with the help of the Federal Ministry of Health, yet have to pay for all the things that truly promote health ourselves.

However, on 6 December 2005, the German Federal Constitutional Court stated in a verdict that statutory health insurance providers must reimburse the costs of alternative medicine for treating life-threatening diseases if they cannot be treated using other methods (BverfG BvR 347/98).

Of course, it is also clear that we had to fight for this right first. In Germany, good lawyers who can successfully guide such processes can be found via the association *Arzt - Recht - Patient*[66].

## Grandchildren

What carries me and my thoughts into the future?

This year another of my grandchildren was born. We were delighted for our children. Life goes on. We are needed in order to pass on our knowledge and experiences. We are happy to be there for our grandchildren with love and patience. We live on in our children and grandchildren. With my granddaughter's birth our souls received a new home. So we have to age healthily. We are determined to do so!

## Light channel therapy

Via a recommendation I came into contact with therapists who had experience in a therapy known as light channel therapy and were now passing on what they had experienced to patients and other therapists.
The aim was to find out where my worries, fears and blockages that were still preventing healing came from with the help of the spiritual world.

We had a session of light channel treatment together. The treatment is a therapy that uses the meridian systems to look for disturbances and/or re-establish connections. The meridians are the channels for life energy, known as the chi in Chinese medicine. If a meridian is interrupted or blocked through illness, shock or something similar, this can be corrected with the help of light channel therapy. One treatment session is often sufficient but several sessions may be carried out if the difficulties are more severe.
The first therapist held my feet loosely in his hands in a way that was familiar to me from craniosacral therapy. The second therapist stood behind me and held my head, my cervical spine and my shoulders; she asked the spiritual helpers for support during the therapy.
We began with the first month of my mother's pregnancy. As I lay on the treatment table what I was doing seemed a little strange. However, the two therapists' calm, secure and professional manner had a very reassuring effect on me.
At the beginning of the treatment I experienced a whole range of sensations. Sometimes a pleasant warmth flowed through me and then suddenly I felt icy cold. The therapists told me what they were feeling, which corresponded to my own sensations. This reassured me.
They asked about each month of the pregnancy. When the question of the fourth month came I suddenly felt extremely restless. It was not until later that I discovered that that was when my mother had

heard the news that my father had been seriously injured and had been taken as a prisoner of war by the Russians.

No information came about the eighth month. Why?

I had not told the therapists that I had been born prematurely at seven months. At the time this meant that the chances of survival were slim. I could still feel the situation within myself, how I was laid aside because no one saw a future for me. After the seventh month was mentioned I was so affected by this that I could hardly think. It was a very emotional situation. My right hand shook even more violently than it had done because of my Parkinson's tremor. I fought! I felt as though the left side of my body was warm and heavy while the right side felt cold and somehow smaller. The therapist identified a blockage in my right knee and right calf.

In my thoughts I was supposed to define myself and command myself to let go of the worries and fears that I was suffering from. I was supposed to say, 'I simply want to let them go.' After some hesitation I was able to do so. It worked! It was wonderful. Gradually the blood began to flow through the right side of my body again and it warmed up right to the tips of my toes. It was more than just pleasant. The therapists thanked the spiritual helpers and the spiritual world for their support.

I did not write my experiences down until a week later. I wanted to have some distance in order to grasp the rational side of it. I was unable to, so I simply wrote it down as I had experienced it.

It was now three weeks after the treatment session. For several days I had felt mild pain and tension in my shoulders similar to the ache sometimes felt after exercise. I could not explain why, as I had not been unusually or especially active.

One morning after my singing bowl therapy I suddenly remembered something from the light channel therapy session. The therapists had said during the treatment that they had noticed that I had put a lot of pressure on myself throughout my life, my youth and my career. However, as I now dealt with my pressure, my fears, my worries and the other strains that were making me ill differently – openly and freely – and repeated again and again to myself 'I want to and I can let everything go', they were gradually symbolically being taken off my shoulders.

It was therefore not surprising that my shoulders and neck now felt relieved and the tension was slowly but surely easing away. Since the treatment I had felt that my circulation was better. My hands and feet now felt pleasantly warm. It had been a long time since I had felt this sensation.


## Dark field microscopy follow-up (II)

In August I had another dark field microscopy follow-up session. I had a blood sample taken at 7.30 a.m., then I had breakfast, and at 9 a.m. was the appointment to discuss the diagnosis.

I was shown the drops of my blood at almost 2000x magnification and was once again surprised at everything that was moving around in there. Yet somehow it was clear even to me, a layperson, that the overall picture had become calmer and more harmonious in comparison to the first examinations.

I now saw uniform, round blood cells that had a beautiful oxygen core; no more of the aggressive viruses and bacteria that attacked and sucked away at the red blood cells. A weak acid crystal and a very small amount of a heavy metal, amalgam, were still recognisable. However, this was no longer a worry; it was actually rather normal and could be corrected with occasional mediation.

The alternative practitioner then said, 'There's nothing more I can do for you, everything's normal!'

What great news. This was something to celebrate.

The timing was great as my wife and I had been invited to celebrate a good friend's birthday with her family and friends in the mountains that evening. Everyone said, 'You two are looking great!' Honestly, after such an event anyone would look good. I felt good too.

I had been more or less torturing myself for a year and a half. With a timer in my pocket I had taken drops, tablets and globules at 20-

minute intervals. I had noticed that some of our friends and family
were very embarrassed to walk through town with me because this
timer kept going off.
But that was unimportant, it had been pain-free – and it had
helped, as I could clearly see.

Once again I had every reason to say THANK YOU!

Now my life felt freer but also less painful, in terms of both physical
and spiritual pain. On many days I was simply happy. Was this
normal? I did not know as I had not experienced it in too long. Yet
my deep consciousness returned gradually and I was now able to
enjoy my new life without a guilty conscience.


## Codex Alimentarius

The Codex Alimentarius was introduced by the United Nations to
provide the world's population with examples of healthy and suitable
food – supposedly. Yet since then exactly the opposite has happened.
It seems to me that the aim of the Codex Alimentarius commission is
to stabilise the pharmaceuticals market.

Here are a few quotes on the topic from Martin Frischknecht's book
*Gesundheit als Chance* (health as an opportunity), translated from the
original German: 'Statements on health regarding the healing effect of
vitamins and other natural materials to prevent disease are to be
prohibited and made punishable. In the future, the definition of what is a
food and what is a medication shall no longer be determined by
governments but by the industry itself. With the help of this law that gives
it power, the pharmaceutical industry will be able to expand its own
market as much as it wishes to.' Later it says: 'The most commonly used
trick of the pharma cartel to discredit vitamins is to attribute some
kind of side effects that damage health to them. The absurd argument
of the pharma politicians is "because vitamins and natural therapies

are so dangerous we must protect the consumer from them." [67]
'A global law that acts as a muzzle in the interest of the pharmaceuticals industry is a protection law to artificially protect a market full of pharmaceutical preparations that have become superfluous and is worth millions. The main cause of this is scientific breakthroughs in vitamin research for almost all widespread diseases. Patients' increasing rejection of conventional medicine and the success of natural medicine are also competition that the pharma cartel must take seriously.' [68]

Finally, M. Frischknecht writes: 'The lethal side effects of pharmaceutical preparations have now taken on such proportions that they have become the fourth most common cause of death worldwide, beaten only by heart attacks, cancer and strokes.' [69, 70]
This should give us something to think about.


## Goji berries

The ways in which I receive pointers are sometimes rather convoluted.
One day I read in a book about the goji berry from China. These small red, very tasty berries have been known in China as *the* healing elixir for around 5000 years.
They contain three times as much vitamin C as oranges. They contain large amounts of minerals and trace elements.
Goji berries can be found all over the world. However, do not be surprised if you read in botanical literature originating from Germany that they are poisonous. [71] The person responsible for this was a researcher named Siebert from Erlangen who, in 1890, classified the plant as poisonous to humans and animals in his thesis for some reason.
Today it is suspected that this was a mix-up. Yet even now people in Germany still copy from him and declare that these wonderful berried are poisonous to humans and animals. Even on the Internet you still

find these incorrect judgements sometimes.

Just one year later, in 1891, a researcher named Schütte proved clearly that the berries from the goji plant are in no way poisonous and – quite the opposite – are highly beneficial for humans.[72]

If you decide to use goji berries you should do so on a daily basis. You will often hear that a good dose for adults is 20 to 30g a day. In China they say a handful of berries a day. Larger people have larger hands and need more; smaller people have smaller hands and therefore take less – a clever method of measurement.[73]

The University of Hong Kong discovered in scientific studies that goji berries help to protect the brain from deteriorating. This is an important discovery for all those suffering from Parkinson's and Alzheimer's disease. I found out that these berries protect against the notorious amyloid peptides that reduce brain performance.

The neurotransmitter dopamine is critical for Parkinson's sufferers. Dopamine is produced in nervous tissue with the help of manganese. Sufficient dopamine levels give us a feeling of relaxation, serenity and harmony. At the same time, our brain and nerve cells produce the happy hormone norepinephrine with the help of enzymes that contain copper. This makes us feel good. However, if there is a lack of manganese and therefore norepinephrine, the stress hormone adrenaline takes action. The results of this are stress, weariness and irritation.

The manganese and copper contained in goji berries are therefore very significant for Parkinson's patients.


## Trampoline

I finally got a trampoline a while ago. Right at the beginning of my journey I had read in the book *Zivilisatoselos*[74] (free from lifestyle diseases) that using a trampoline was strongly recommended. At first I was afraid that I would not be able to use it at all, as I constantly

felt dizzy and had difficulty moving my legs. The idea of getting my
own trampoline was forgotten but remained it the back of my mind.
Now I had put the idea into practice and was excited. However, it
had been difficult to find the right trampoline for me. After many
tests and offers I chose a particularly soft trampoline.
I had begun my search carefully and warily. Luckily I found someone with a
great deal of specialist knowledge at a trampoline shop who advised me
very well. As I tested the many different types of trampoline I became more
and more confident after just a few minutes.
Today I have my own trampoline at home; I use it every day and feel
much better. I think that such a device is really very helpful for all
Parkinson's patients.
Please at least give it a try!
As you bounce the vertebral disks achieve a good vertical position and
the spine and the surrounding muscles are strengthened.
The lymph drainage effect is especially significant for Parkinson's
sufferers. The lymphatic circulation is sped up considerably by the
gentle rhythmic movement. The neuro-muscular system of channels is
activated, which has a particularly positive effect on brain
performance. The increase in oxygen through improved circulation is
more than 60 percent higher than when running.[75]
Through the natural balance and coordination work you become
more sure footed. It is easier to lift your feet. I also felt that it
made implementing the brain's commands to the leg muscles
easier. The metabolism is stimulated and the joints benefit because
the joint cartilage is provided with liquid more effectively. 'With the
same oxygen consumption, the greatest acceleration of the body
(as an indicator of the work put in) when bouncing on a trampoline
is up to 68 percent higher than when running. In other words,
much more is achieved with a given amount of oxygen when
rebounding than on a treadmill.'[76]

The exact product names and the names and addresses for the
products I have used and suggestions given in this book are

available from my independent, non-profit self-help organisation, Selbsthilfeorganisation elementares Wissen e.V. Information about the organisation can be found at the end of the book.


## A circle closes

After all these years, my thoughts returned to 2001 and 2002. I remembered my initial feelings about my Parkinson's disease. Although at that time my disease had not yet been confirmed, my daily life did not feel the same as before. My concentration had weakened noticeably and I felt an unusually pressing need to go out into nature. The slightest ray of sunshine compelled me to leave my desk immediately to enjoy the sun, the light and the air. Unfortunately, my diary did not allow me to do this. I felt that the decision to keep working was wrong but I could not get past the feeling of responsibility that was so ingrained in me. It was not until 2003 that I discovered that I might be suffering from Parkinson's disease, which was confirmed at the DKD in 2004.

I remembered my mental block from the early stages of my disease, which was particularly severe when the sun shone. Back then I could not understand this.

By 'chance' I heard about Jakob Lorber (1800–1864). He is considered a pioneer of heliopathy, the knowledge of the powers of healing stored in sunlight. In his book *The Healing Power of Sunlight* he describes the dual nature of sunlight, a phenomenon that biophysicists are only just beginning to understand and measure in this form.

The energies carried in sunlight are tied directly to the carrier substances in the plant, mineral and animal world. These elements of sunlight strengthen the soul and can promote the healing effects in the long term.

More than 150 years ago, Jakob Lorber wrote in his theses that there is a pure energy contained in the sun's light that has a significant relationship to the human soul. This pure sun energy is of elementary importance for the human soul and therefore human health.

When we feel ill and lacking in energy after long periods of grey weather, stress or other strains, our souls have, according to Lorber, taken energy from our organs. An unnatural process occurs in our bodies, which is responsible for different kinds of disease.

Too little sunlight makes us ill.

The physical symptoms of disease are an expression of the state of our souls. We need the sun's light for all of the vital processes in our bodies, especially for healing. Each cell is nourished by this light energy. We are therefore able to absorb all the substances which, according to Jakob Lorber, make up our souls via sunlight and to correct a lack of energy.

The communication that takes place between the biophotons in sunlight and the biophotons in the human body takes place at the cell level and can be measured today. The sunlight penetrates the cell to its core in order to supply organs and nerves. Biophysicists can prove these things scientifically.

It is often underestimated how important exposure to sunlight is for us, even as children. If the body already does not get enough sun when we are young this can allow many diseases to develop. Of course we are often told that due to excessive $CO_2$ and the hole in the ozone layer UV radiation is becoming ever more intense. This is entirely correct. However, here, as in all cases, the following applies: the dose makes the poison.

The human body needs the sun as it is one of the main sources of energy. To put it simply, as humans crave good water, they also crave the sun. If this energy that our souls need so desperately is lacking we cannot heal.

Today I understand my strong yearning to go into the sun, to go outdoors and to go out into nature during the first few years of my disease.

If we look back through human history we find traces of the Greek city of Heliopolis.

The 'city of the sun' was famous for its temple in which sunlight was split up into spectral colours in order to heal various diseases. Goethe and Einstein also refer to the power of the sun's energy that is essential for us. This is sunlight and it remains our most important source of nourishment!


What lives in me?

The knowledge that around 70 to 80 billion cells in our bodies control our lives is hard to imagine. To give a better idea, 100000 cells are around the size of a pinhead. However, that we are able, just with our thoughts, to initiate energy frequencies in our cells that can be both positive (a state of health) and harmful, even to the point where they cause diseases that destroy our bodies, is absolutely fascinating. DNA is packed into chromosomes in the nucleus of each of these approximately 80 million cells. When DNA mutates, there is a lack of free radical scavengers and vitamins. More oxygen is burned. This is a simplified version of what happens, but it still describes the path to all diseases. Our cells contain collagen, a gelatine-like substance, which acts as a light conductor and produces photons. Studies have shown that these photons change in neurons in cell cultures and send out light and energy from the chakra system. At the same time, the meridians form a kind of fibre bundle, similar to a fibre optic cable. These processes have been visibly documented by the scientist Donald Ingber and were clearly demonstrated by the biologist Dr Armin Koroknay in a lecture at the first Appenzeller Health Congress in 2009 in Schwellbrunn in Switzerland. German scientists are now also able to make meridian and acupuncture points visible using biophoton photography. For many years these terms, which originate from the Far East, were pushed aside and branded esoteric beliefs. Yet these points really exist. They are visible to us and can be measured by researchers. Dr Koroknay also spoke about the most amazing aspects of the body in his exciting lecture.
Everything that we think, eat and drink – essentially how we live – has a long-term effect on our cells. Frequencies from light and sound

develop and influence the way in which DNA reads genes, as if a concert were taking place in each cell and uniting with the light of the meridians. It is as if every second 150 million videos are being played at the same time. For this reason, the cell biologist Bruce Lipton talks about intelligent cells. We are what we believe! Back in Antiquity, Hippocrates of Cos, a scholar from Asclepius and one of the most important figures in the history of medicine (Rod of Asclepius), recognised a simple yet crucial principle as to how we should lead our lives: 'Let food be our medicine and heal us with nutrition.'

I create my own reality and my environment, how I experience it and how I construct it. I am what I think, eat and feel. The soul, mind and body are feelings, thoughts, food and drink. I think, therefore I am! Everything happens through the energies in the food that I eat and through the energies of my lifestyle. My mind is stronger than my genes.

Ancient teachings on the spirt of plants and on alchemy were put into practice by the mystic doctor Paracelsus (Theophrast von Hohenheim, 1493–1541). Paracelsus supported the effectiveness of his medications through the power of the mind.

It was not until centuries later that Dr Samuel Hahnemann was able to give us his frequency patterns defined by homeopathic globules. In his research back in the 1980s, Dr Wolfgang Ludwig (1927–2004) was able to prove the effect of the homeopathic globules through measurable energy. Nowadays, practitioners who are sufficiently informed commonly use bioresonance devices in their medical diagnoses. These devices are able to show information about thousands of the patient's genes in a matter of seconds. These genes provide the code for essential enzymes and can be influenced by changes in homeopathic frequencies. These frequencies can recognise and influence these sensations, even very small ones.

In the normal state of harmony waves are strengthened; if there is conflict, on the other hand, the wave is reduced until it disappears.

For this reason, we should honestly strive for harmony in our lives as a whole, in our daily lives and in our families, and we should learn to allow an integral consciousness.

The intuition of our guts, hearts and heads determines how we process our feelings. Diseases are partly a manifestation of forgotten frequency patterns or information that have a considerable effect on our potential for health. We should be ever more shaped by unconditional love, as it does not allow anything harmful in. We can decide.

The human being of the future should be loving, or he will cease to be at all! To allow us to live in this duality, we must no longer say 'either… or…'; instead we should allow 'both… and…'. This is tolerance and gives us freedom.

Do not evaluate anything any longer. This is my new motto for a healthy life. Let us finally separate ourselves from the old ways of thinking that have been fed to us and that limit and restrict our lives![77]


## Decision

According to Clemens Kuby, constant uncertainty in the healthcare system requires each individual to gain their own skills in healing and health.[78]

According to many doctors and a large proportion of the general public, Parkinson's disease cannot be cured.

What do you want?

Do you want to take 'wonderful' medication, along with its harmful side effects, until the very last day? Or do you choose natural medication with research into the cause? The latter can take many months, but be patient, as it gets better every day.

Unfortunately, in my experience, some Parkinson's sufferers would rather take a daily cocktail of chemical medication to slow down the disease and ignore the sometimes long-term natural opportunities for healing. What I hear is 'It's too hard; it takes too long,' and similar answers.

Please consider that only nature can give you the chance to live healthily and free from problems again over the coming years. We make our own destiny, so the saying goes. I have made my decision, as I can only finally become healthy again with natural medicine.

As of 2011, I can say that I am healed.
It was a long journey that has paid off for me in many ways. After I identified the causes of my Parkinson's disease, thanks to my new way of life I was immediately able to see an improvement due to the natural medications and my energy-giving meditation. I moved forward slowly but surely.

At the same time, other illnesses that I had had all my life disappeared, such as the rheumatic problems I had had since my childhood, the headaches and disc problems, my sensitivity to the weather, the pains in my knees and feet, the liver, kidney and prostate problems, and much more. I was able to experience this in my own body.
True healing covers the whole person and not just one organ or one part of the body. Or, as Clemens Kuby puts it, when we understand that we are spiritual beings, our being gains another dimension.[79]


## Last chance

Sometimes a person who is looking for a cure can be confused by the options that are available. They can be unsure. They cannot and do not want to try everything. In this case, it helps to take some time out, to meditate or to pray in order to decide how to proceed. You have to learn to differentiate! In this context, I remember the story of a priest who sits on the roof of his church during a terrible flood and prays to the man upstairs. A rescue team with a boat comes to rescue him, but he turns down their help, saying 'God will help me.' The next day, the water has risen even further. The rescue team comes past again, but

the priest simply says, 'You can go on past, God will help me.' A few
hours later, the water has risen so high that the priest is struggling to
cling on to the steeple. The rescue team's helicopter comes to help him,
but even now he says, 'Fly on by, God will help me.' When the next
wave of flood water comes he disappears. Standing before God he
asks, 'God, why didn't you help me?' And God answers, 'What more
can I do? I sent you rescuers three times!'


## Recognise your opportunities

Check every form of help that is offered to you – whether it is
medication or therapy. Never fall back into a pattern of thinking or an
educational pattern or old beliefs.
Become free in your thoughts, as any honest form of help that happens
through love and compassion is the right one, even if it is only a small part in
the large mosaic of our health.
Without this small piece, our health is not complete and this can lead
to another breakdown. A large number of big and small puzzle pieces
(therapies) can have a crucial effect on making us healthy again.
Look for them! These solutions exist! Ask for them! You are sure to
receive an answer! Do not leave out any piece of the puzzle until the
picture of your health and your happiness is complete again!
I wish you all patience when implementing therapies; patience with
yourselves, love and compassion for you and your loved ones, for
family, friends and therapists, and for your personal peace in
reconciliation.

*Peace – Frieden – Salam – Pace – Schalom – Shanti – Paix*


## My thanks

I planned to set up an independent, non-profit self-help organisation.
First and foremost, I intended to use the donations to support
individuals in individual projects, but I also wanted people looking for

help to be able to come to the organisation.

After my odyssey over the past few years I was forced to see that almost no one can really help. They either cannot or are not allowed to or do not want to. The possibilities of natural medicine or homeopathic medicine or complementary medicine are not taken seriously, despite many positive publications in a few courageous journals or in positive critical television programmes.
For this reason, I wanted to provide information and research the causes of Parkinson's disease and this was to be the aim of my self-help organisation.
Furthermore, I wanted to establish an award for individuals or universities, institutions, or research groups who had the courage to publish new findings and were not afraid to make complementary, integrative medicine available to us patients through their scientific findings. It was my intention that this innovative work should enable recognition and support to be gathered from general practitioners, health insurance providers and public health authorities.
My concept included finding people who did not just provide hope but would also really and directly help to organise the essentials for those who needed help.
Lay people are allowed to share their experiences and the possibilities of alternative forms of medicine in self-help groups and organisations. It is important to ensure that the money that is donated genuinely fulfils its intended purpose. The administrative work was to be carried out by committed individuals; the costs were to be kept to a minimum.

After I had considered a self-help group for several days, it became clear that I needed a name that expressed the help on offer simply and effectively, and that would be understood internationally. I meditated and suddenly I had it. I had found the term I was looking for: *elementares Wissen* = elementary knowledge.
Now it was time to put my idea into practice!

I was determined to set up a strong, trustworthy self-help organisation that would live up to its name with solidity and solidarity. I would make sure of it personally.

*If I had only one prayer, it would be THANK YOU.* (Meister Eckehart)

# Part II
# New perspectives
# on causes and therapies

# Possible causes of Parkinson's disease


## 1. Soul/psyche

Mental block (see anthroposophic therapies below),
unprocessed experiences from childhood,
traumatic situations experienced by mother during pregnancy

## 2. Body

Diseases of organs, such as liver diseases,
lymphatic diseases, particular diseases of the lymph nodes
in the head,
diseases of the pancreas, lungs, spleen, intestine, gallbladder, kidneys, small
intestine, large intestine, skin, etc.,
lack of vitamins and minerals

## 3. Impurities and infections

Intestinal fungi, viruses, bacteria, leeches, Lyme disease, mutated
fungi/camouflaged candida or similar in the blood,
accumulations of the same in the brain, etc.

## 4. Overacidification

Overacidification of the affected organs and bodily fluids such as the liver,
kidneys, skin, blood, etc.,
as a consequence of overacidification of the whole body

## 5. Toxification

Side effects of medications, vaccinations,
environmental toxins,
heavy metals,
amalgam, mercury, palladium and similar,
insecticides, pesticides, wood protector,
softening agents in cosmetics and plastics,

aluminium, manganese and lead,
carbon monoxide,
diesel particles,
domestic toxins, formaldehyde and more,
toxins from food,
medications, in particular antipsychotics or calcium channel blockers

## 6. Lifestyle

Poor nutrition,
harmful foods, glutamate, aspartame, etc.,
harmful E numbers (additives approved by the EU), fizzy drinks, processed meats, etc.,
unhealthy lifestyle, hectic lifestyle, stress,
cigarettes, etc.,
alcohol,
fast food, junk food

## 7. Brain/mind

Multiple-system atrophy = degeneration of the structures and systems of the central nervous system (CNS) due to, for example: stroke,
meningitis,
brain tumour,
bleeding in the brain in the substantia nigra (dark brain matter in the midbrain),
drug consumption,
injections of pethidine analogues (e.g. drug substitutes),
Creutzfeldt-Jakob disease,
lack of minerals,
lack of vitamins,
overacidification,
heavy metals (e.g. amalgam),
harmful blood terrain (fungi and mutated fungi, viruses, bacteria)

## 8. ADD/ADHD

E.g. in childhood,
can also be caused by lasting effects of medications

## 9. Consequences of accidents

Falls or knocks, impacts to the head, etc.,
even seemingly simple falls where the spine was damaged which may have
happened several years before,
sports injuries, risks from sport, etc.

## 10. Environment

Geopathic features such as:
water veins, earth radiation, Hartmann grids, etc.,
electro smog,
magnetic fields,
radio masts,
noise pollution, motorways, airports, cities, etc.,
light pollution in cities

# Possible therapies for Parkinson's disease

The following suggestions are based on my findings and experiences collected while suffering from this disease between 2003 and 2010. First of all, it is important to recognise and acknowledge with love and thanks that this disease, like all other diseases, is a signal and a reaction to your previous lifestyle.
Seek with confidence. Expand your knowledge with determination in order to become fully healthy again.

If faith can move mountains, then it is the faith in our own powers.

List of possible therapies

The following therapies are individual components, like those of a mosaic or puzzle, that we can put together to enable us to lead a normal, healthy life again:

1 Deacidification of the body
2 An alkaline lifestyle
3 Minerals according to Dr Schüßler's method and antioxidants
4 Vitamins and supplementary preparations
5 Blood health
6 Intestinal health
7 Rudolf Breuss' treatment
8 Health in the environment and the home
9 Healing stone therapy
10 Physiotherapy
11 Meridian therapy
12 Craniosacral therapy
13 Singing bowl therapy
14 Consciousness therapy with Bach flower remedies
15 Heavy metal detoxification
16 Meditation
17 Psychotherapy
18 Eating and living healthily
19 Relationships
20 Maria Treben's therapy
21 Water crystals
22 Healing water
23 Hildegard therapy
24 Rechtsregulat
25 Homeopathic therapy
26 Anthroposophic therapy
27 Lymph therapy

28 Aslan therapy
29 Horst Krone's therapy
30 Vibration and elementary energy
31 Order therapies
32 Trampolining
33 Oxygen therapy
34 Permanent acupuncture and other forms of acupuncture
35 Chelation therapy
36 Indian healing plants
37 Healing animal venoms
38 Copper
39 Frankincense
40 Music and dance
41 Paranormal surgery and trance medicine
42 Spiritual astrology and astromedicine
43 Early diagnosis – the best therapy

[For more suggestions and tips see part III, chap. What really helps us (work sheet 4).]

The most important thing is to create your own overall concept based on the possible therapies listed above, some of which are very different from one another, and to follow it consistently. The body, soul and mind must all be treated equally.

It would be possible to write entire books on the subjects of each of the short chapters here. For this reason, the information has been condensed considerably and is only intended as a starting point. The content that I present is usually not quoted word for work but is summarised and supplemented by my own experiences and findings. I therefore ask that you consult the literature mentioned and find details and exact information there.

Finally, I strongly recommend that you find out whether your disease can be recognised as a disability by your local authorities. In Germany, for example, Parkinson's and Alzheimer's disease can be recognised as a disability due to the effects on aspects such as mobility, entitling sufferers to hold a disability badge. Please contact the appropriate authorities in your country to find out about the options available to you.

# The therapy mosaic

## 1. Deacidification of the body

What causes overacidification?

Overacidification is essentially a consequence of our civilisation: too much of everything, too much fat, too many sweet things, stress, fast food, etc. Overacidification of the body restricts crucial processes in the metabolism or stops them completely, as the overacidification takes up all of the vitamins and minerals. We need to realise that acids are constantly forming in our bodies. It is a wonder that they are able to neutralise or even eliminate them.

Uric acid is produced by the metabolic breakdown of animal protein and by cell decay.
Acetic acid is produced during the metabolic breakdown of carbohydrates and fat when the breakdown is incomplete.
Lactic acid is produced when muscles are highly active, such as during strenuous physical activity and various sports, from weight training to marathon running.
Sulphuric acid is produced during decay in the intestine but also in the metabolic breakdown of pork.
Keto acid is produced during the breakdown of fat from fat deposits.
Hydrochloric acid is produced when we have an upset stomach (stress, aggravation) and when we have a severe alkali deficiency.
Oxalic acid is produced when the body consumes cocoa, asparagus, tomatoes, spinach, chard or rhubarb.
Tannic acid is produced by black tea or coffee.
Nitric acid is produced by curing salt or by calcium nitrate used in the food industry, corresponding E numbers and carbon dioxide (e.g. carbonated water), acetic acid, etc.[1]

Each acid by itself is problematic. Disastrous consequences occur when one acid comes into contact with another acid or with additives, including legal additives that are apparently not harmful. We must inform ourselves about these processes. Chemists call the combination of sulphuric acid, nitric acid and hydrochloric acid 'aqua regia', literally 'king's water'. It is the only chemical compound that can dissolve gold.[2] It is the most corrosive known substance in the world. It is amazing that our bodies can tolerate this combination of acids in small quantities, therefore we should not flood them with uncontrolled doses of it. This makes us ill!

Overacidification can begin to take place in the womb due to the mother's diet and lifestyle (such as eating large quantities or ice cream or chocolate). Later the wrong kinds of food and sweet products (in the sense of industrial sugars) that cause an acidic chemical reaction in our bodies add to the effect. This overacidification immediately destroys the minerals and vitamins that we get from our food. This leads to a lack of vitamins, minerals and water, infections, rheumatism, osteoporosis, and over 40 different lifestyle diseases, including Parkinson's disease.
We must stay away from certain kinds of food and other substances to deacidify the body, as they do not benefit us. These include coffee, alcohol, tobacco and nicotine, but also meat – especially pork and processed meats – and cheese. I believe that carbon dioxide in carbonated drinks is a particular problem as these drinks are so widely advertised. The consumer has no idea that they are consuming something harmful. The same applies to sweets, ice cream, chocolate and the like.

Natural medicine distinguishes between:
1. Latent overacidification, where all connective tissue and organs are flooded with acids.
2. Compensated overacidification, where the excretory organs are permanently in overdrive, leading to inflammation and catarrh.
3. Decompensated overacidification, where the blood, tissue and cells can no longer cope with the flood of acids. This leads to increasing toxification of the organs and tissue and causes chronic illness. This broadly corresponds to the level of illness in Germany, for example with regard to rheumatic diseases and many other diseases.

Helpful drinking pure high-quality water (pH value of over 7.0),
getting rid of infections, changing diet, purifying the liver, and
activating the kidneys.


## 2. An alkaline lifestyle

First of all, the following are to be strictly avoided: regularly eating
canteen food, eating at irregular intervals, eating hastily, fried
products such as chips and crisps, milk products (except cream),
meat, processed meats, alcohol, sweet things such as biscuits and
chocolate.
Instead, it is essential to choose food that contains many alkaline
substances. This includes all types of lettuce, herbs, sweet and sour
fruit and vegetables (except Brussels sprouts and artichoke bottoms),
and dried fruits that do not contain sulphites.

Do not doubt!
The absence of doubts will allow you to fulfil your wish of becoming
healthy again quicker. After a few weeks of consciously living an
alkaline lifestyle and seeing a noticeable improvement in your
symptoms you can attempt to prepare yourself for the future with
regards to your diet.

Today I ensure that two thirds of each meal are alkaline, such as
vegetables, potatoes and salad, while a third is non-alkaline, such
as fish or cheese.
Alcohol such as wine or beer should initially be avoided for one to two
years and later only consumed in small quantities, if at all, and along
with at least the same quantity of water in order to neutralise its
effects. The same applies to coffee. In some countries coffee is always
served with water. Spirits should be completely banned from your life
forever!
Stress must be avoided or neutralised. This is best done through
meditation, relaxation exercises, autogenic training or yoga. This

allows the mind and body to find peace. I find it ideal and practice it every day.

The alkaline lifestyle begins with a urine pH measurement in the morning. The pH value should be between 6.5 and 7.0. If it is below this it can be easily corrected with an alkaline lifestyle. This is certainly not a quick fix, but you have to consider that it has taken overacidification years to ruin the body.
First we begin with alkaline baths, initially only once a week. After around three weeks this can be increased to two baths a week. These baths are truly the easiest and, at the same time, most effective way of managing overacidification. In addition, before the bath I use a Baunscheidt roller (available from specialist shops) on my whole body.
I buy alkaline bath salts from health food shops from brands such as Aurica. There are many other brands available, such as Meine Base or Bullrichs basische Bäder. Put about four tablespoons, usually more, in the bath water, which should have a temperature around 38°C, until you reach a pH value of 8.5 to 9.0. This high-quality alkaline water mirrors the amniotic fluid in the womb and is considered optimal.
The amount of alkaline salt or powder required depends on the quality of the tap water and the content of the tub; the amounts recommended by the manufacturer are usually too small. When you take your first bath you should measure the pH value exactly with pH test strips. The bath should last at least one hour but can last longer. So that I do not get too cold or bored I scrub my body with a rough brush and a hard flannel. I do this in the direction of the excretory organs, i.e. from the knees down to the tips of the toes (natural medicine calls the skin our largest organ and the feet our 'auxiliary kidneys' when removing acid), from the knees up toward the genitals, from the stomach and chest to the armpits, from the back down to the anus and from the head down to the neck, chest or armpits. Do not forget to do behind your ears.
Over time you will develop your own ritual.

Two times a day I drink an alkaline drink, such as one from the brand
Dr Jacobs. Every day I eat one to two teaspoons of Wurzelkraft (a
mixture of different alkaline fruits, roots, herbs, etc.) and drink
several cups of alkaline herbal tea or the 7x7 herbal tea from Dr Peter
Jentschura[3] or a similar drink. This procedure provides the perfect
support for my efforts.
With regard to fluids, you should drink at least 1 litre of herbal tea
and 1 to 1.5 litres of spring water and/or water energised with
healing stones every day. In the summer months when it is very hot
these amounts should be increased accordingly.
After the alkaline bath you should not dry yourself but only dab away
the moisture or allow the moisture from the alkaline bath to dry on
your skin. After a while the alkaline baths can be complemented with
alkaline foot baths, alkaline socks, etc. From day to day, an alkaline
nasal rinse with alkaline bath salt is particularly helpful.
For patients with diseases of the brain, such as Parkinson's disease,
the cavities of the head must be rinsed regularly, i.e. two to three
times a day, and cleaned by gargling or, if required, inhaling. This
also helps to prevent colds as bacteria cannot settle in an alkaline
space.
You should drink large amounts of water – good still water such as
Evian or Volvic, enriched with healing stones and $H_2O_2$ when possible.
This increases the water's energy and is highly beneficial for the cells
and organs.

Nowadays my wife and I also pay particular attention to what we eat.
Ready meals and pre-cooked food, whether it comes from the freezer
or is left over from the day before, are taboos for us because all of the
vitamins are lost when food is reheated. Rudolf Breuss once gave a
good illustration of this. He compares a person's health to the roof of a
house. If, after a heavy storm (disease), ten tiles (vitamins and
minerals) are missing and you only replace eight of them, whether it is
due to carelessness or costs, one day you will not have any tiles left on
the roof.

If that is not convincing enough, Rudolf Breuss also has a scientific experiment concerning reheated food to hand. Researchers carried out the following experiment using 150 mice. 50 mice were given freshly cooked food. For another 50, the food was cooled for 20 minutes and then reheated. For the remaining 50, the food was cooled for 5 hours and then reheated and given to them.
Within one month, everything went terribly for the third group of 50 mice. One mouse lost all of the hair on its body within two hours and died two hours later. In other mice a foot, the tail or the ears died off. Others died without any external indications of the reason. They were then dissected and it was discovered that their oesophagus had deteriorated and become separated or that their kidneys had stopped growing. In this group of 50 mice it took one month until the last one died. In the group whose food was only cooled for 20 minutes and then reheated, it took 3 months before they all died in the same way. The first group of 50 mice that received freshly cooked food were all still completely healthy after 3 months!

When we are hungry it is a sign that cells have died and want to be replaced by fresh food. However, if we eat reheated or recooked food, which is therefore lacking in vitamins, in the long term these cells are not replaced. This means that reheated food is not just useless but can actually be harmful.[4]
Frozen fresh red berries, spinach and herbs, on the other hand, are recommended, as long as they are organic. It is particularly important to watch out for any artificial additives in food. People are organic beings and cannot tolerate chemical substances. Inorganic, artificial additives, flavour enhancers and preservatives seriously harm our lives.
So make sure you watch out for E numbers when you go shopping![5]
Products without barcodes from the industry are often more beneficial!


## 3. Minerals according to Dr Schüßler's method and antioxidants
The German doctor Dr Wilhelm Heinrich Schüßler (1821–1898) was very controversial in his time. He studied in Paris, Prague and

Berlin.[6] It was not until he was 52 years old that he published his
biochemical healing methods in the *Allgemeine homöopathische
Zeitung* newspaper with which, he claimed, he could heal almost any
disease using 12 different mineral salts.
Since, at this time, homeopathy already had around 4000
homeopathic substances, this greatly simplified medication was
highly suspicious and was not recognised. His colleagues accused
Schüßler of damaging their reputation and called the Schüßler salts
manure.
Wilhelm Schüßler did not live to see his salts recognised and promoted. It
was only during the First World War and in the 1930s that his products began
to be tolerated and later accepted as a welcome, inexpensive form of
therapy.

From today's perspective, Schüßler salts provide a solid method of
balancing out our depleted mineral levels in general and especially for
Parkinson's sufferers. The starting point for this is to be prepared to
want to change your own lifestyle and to lead a healthy, conscious life.
One of the forms in which Parkinson's sufferers should take the fine
minerals is in the form of Dr Schüßler's salts. Schüßler's idea was to
combine an alkaline and an acidic element in each tablet or globule.
For example, in the Calcium phosphoricum (calcium phosphate) salt,
calcium is the alkaline element and phosphorus is the acidic element.
In this way our bodies, strengthened by this combination, do not have
to combine the individual elements.

The following salts are recommended to support Parkinson's patients:
Calcium phosphoricum no. 2; Magnesium phosphoricum no. 7; Silicea
no. 11.[6, 7]
I myself have taken the following combination: Calcium
phosphoricum no. 2, Kalium chloratum no. 4 , Silicea no. 11, Ferrum
phosporicum no. 3, Kalium phosphoricum no. 5, Magnesium
phosphoricum no. 7.[8]
My experiences come from long term use but are very positive. I felt

the beneficial effects of Magnesium phosphoricum and Kalium phosphoricum within just a few days. Later, with the exception of no. 5, which I took until 2010, I exchanged the salts listed above for others based on how I felt.

You should seek advice on the strength, types and doses to take from an experienced therapist. In principle these salts are a fantastic method for correcting the mineral levels in the body. However, there have been reports that some of the minerals in Schüßler salts are made of synthetic substances. This is considered disadvantageous for those with heart disease and high blood pressure.
Therefore, make sure you pay attention to the manufacturer and discuss this with your pharmacist and change if necessary. The manufacturer of my Schüßler salts uses potato starch as a binding agent instead of the usual lactose. This can be very beneficial for diabetics as otherwise they are normally unable to take Schüßler salts.

As we are constantly exposed to electro smog and electromagnetic radiation, our bioelectric field needs more of the minerals that we are already lacking. A permanent lack of minerals is already pre-programmed into us. Furthermore, most people have various metals in their mouths in the form of bridges, crows, fillings, implants, etc. This alone causes minerals to be trapped and used up in the mouth. This can cause mineral deficiency.
These causes can be partially compensated for by Schüßler products, but there is often a lack of knowledge of the appropriate amounts. I determine my own course of therapy with my pendulum but there is also good literature available on the subject.
I also take selenium in the permitted dosage in alternation with other supplements, such as chlorella algae, AfA algae, ginkgo, folic acid or coenzyme Q10. I alternate calcium, selenium, manganese, magnesium, chromium, zinc, iodine, etc. in appropriate doses with other preparations such as omega 3 fatty acids, wheat germ oil,

evening primrose oil or gamma-linoleic acid. In terms of important
natural antioxidants, aronia berries, schisandra berries and goji
berries are recommended.

*Important note:* It is better not to use combination preparations of
minerals and vitamins, as the vitamins often cancel out the effect of the
minerals in the body. For example, when selenium is taken at the same
time as vitamin C it is removed from the body without any effect.
These products are usually expensive and unfortunately useless. For
this reason, I consciously separate my intake, for example by taking
vitamins in the morning and minerals at midday.

## 4. Vitamins and supplementary preparations

Most people intend to eat vitamin-rich food. However, unfortunately,
nowadays our food rarely contains the required quantities of vitamins
that it used to 50 years ago. This means that we are forced not only
to supplement these essential vitamins but also to slowly bring up the
vitamin levels that have been depleted through disease.

The following recommendations and recommended frequencies (e.g.
'every day') are based on the first few years of my natural therapies.
Today, now that I am healed, I use much smaller quantities. The
most important vitamins for Parkinson's patients are all B vitamins,
along with vitamin C, D and E.

I initially took vitamin C in large doses in the form of natural, pure
vitamin C.
*Important note:* It is essential that you only use natural vitamin C
that is produced, for example, from acerola cherries, rose hips or
oranges. Do not take the synthetic vitamin sold as vitamin C (ascorbic
acid). The recommend doses of this synthetic substance can make
you ill, particularly if you have heart problems. I take vitamin E every
day, such as in the form of highly beneficial wheat germ oil. It is also

available as capsules.

The sun helps with vitamin D. The tablets that you can buy do not contain vitamin D but simply support the body's ability to produce it. However, in principle we only need sunlight. Allowing sunlight to shine on your face and hands for half an hour each day is sufficient. Certain studies state that using sunscreen with a protection factor of eight or higher prevents vitamin D from being formed. In medicine the name vitamin D is currently considered incorrect, as vitamin D is not a vitamin but a hormone.

Once a year I do a 60 day course of therapy to stabilise my liver with liver vitamins. Today I do a similar thing with the vitamins mentioned above. However, I use the natural active agents in milk thistle, artichoke, dandelion and other plants. Lapacho, a bark powder from Brazil that I took in 2009 and 2010 to support my body's defences, supports the liver and lymph nodes and has a generally detoxifying effect. Lapacho strengthens the immune system and is capable of developing antibodies itself.
If, for example, the liver is only able to fulfil its job as a filtering and detoxifying organ in a limited capacity and invading microbes and fungi are allowed to multiply out of control and destroy the intestinal flora, the lapacho defence system takes over. Lapacho contains rare mineral salts and trace elements. It has been shown to be particularly helpful for Parkinson's disease, diabetes, inflammation in the large intestine, rheumatism, inflammation of the prostate and other conditions. American and British researchers have used lapacho to treat different kinds of cancer since the 1960s and it has promoted healing. I believe this to be highly recommended!

You should also carry out a course of therapy to cleanse your liver and remove gall and liver stones once a year. Either use Dr Clark's[9] very simple methods or those described by Martin Frischknecht[10].
Once a year I do the kidney cleansing course designed by Rudolf

Breuss over a period of three weeks.[11] This can easily be done at the same time and requires comparatively little effort.
I do the Tibetan garlic cure mentioned earlier (see part I, Garlic cure) once or twice a year in alternation with the courses mentioned above.

*Tip:* Do not stick to your doctor or alternative practitioner regardless. If you sense uncertainty, particularly if you are met by outright rejections or unexplained reasoning, the time has come to find out who else can help.
For me, it was changing doctors and practitioners, and hearing new and sometimes different opinions that helped move forward down the path to healing. You just need to be brave! Always formulate your problems and wishes clearly. Do not allow yourself to be satisfied by being told 'Just take this and come back in two weeks.'
This will not help you because it means that your doctor or practitioner is still looking for a solution themselves. These two weeks are lost time. You do not have time for that! Do not allow yourself to be dazzled by diagnoses like 'idiopathic Parkinson's disease'. This may sound nice but essentially says nothing more than that your doctor does not really know whether you are actually suffering from Parkinson's disease or not.


## 5. Blood health

Keeping our blood healthy should be one of our main concerns. It is crucial to recognise fungi, heavy metals, leeches, bacteria and viruses in the blood at an early stage. The best results are achieved with dark field microscopy where the blood is examined at 2000x magnification. Anyone who has ever seen on a monitor all the acid crystals, trichomonads, mutated candida fungi, heavy metals and other things whizzing around in a drop of blood knows that the blood is one of nature's greatest wonders. A radionic test can be carried out afterwards to determine the Parkinson's factor. Unfortunately, this science is rarely represented in Germany (this has to do with events that happened during unpleasant parts of German history). However, courageous alternative practitioners such as Ekkehard Scheller are still carrying out research and helping people with it.[12]

Here are just a few examples of the unbelievable pollution of our blood caused by heavy metals. It has now been discovered that in patients with Parkinson's disease these heavy metals accumulate in the brain, damaging its nerves. In most cases, as it was in mine, the heavy metals in the brain are trapped in fungi, making it impossible for the instructions transmitted by the nerves in the brain to be implemented, for example to walk or to speak. Furthermore, the fungi mean that they cannot be reached with the usual methods to detoxify the body of heavy metals.
Accumulations of heavy metals can have many causes, such as pesticides and insecticides, wood protector, tattoos, and vaccinations. All of these substances contain heavy metals, for example mercury. The main cause is amalgam which, for example, is
used in fillings for teeth. Amalgam consists of:
58% mercury
16% tin
19% silver
15% copper and nickel, also known as high copper amalgam.

Heavy metals in the mouth affect the liver, kidneys and brain due to salivation alone. These effects are increased by food which is too hot or too acidic. This leads to gradual toxification with mild to severe symptoms such as discomfort, kidney failure, nerve damage, brain damage, a weakened immune system, inflammation, skin irritation and psychological conditions such as depression.
We do not perceive this toxification directly. It develops within us over decades.
However, all other diseases are also recognisable in our blood at an early stage. Dark field microscopy allows diseases in the blood

to be recognised that have not yet made themselves apparent in
the body through complaints and pains.
In the last few years before my Parkinson's disease manifested
itself openly, from around 2000 onwards, I felt burning tears in
my eyes. This could be when I was reading, watch television or in
a meeting and began to happen more and more frequently. If I
drove for an extended period of time I often had to stop and let
someone else take over. I simply could not see anymore. Was
this overacidification? The signs pointed to uveitis, an
autoimmune disease. Around five years ago, before going blind,
my mother had also suffered constant pain due to similar acidic,
irritating tears that affected her retinas. No one could help her.
She was constantly being treated by different doctors and
optometrists. Of course I was scared that over time my disease
would take me down the same path as my mother.
Due to the dark field microscopy examinations, the treatment that
stemmed from them, the lifestyle I practice, and other things, these
symptoms have also disappeared completely.

People need to be considered as a whole. Everyone should practice this
themselves. Know yourself, love yourself and accept yourself! This
strong, unshakeable intention alone is often enough to influence the
over 40,000 pure memory cells in our organic hearts so positively that
we can heal. The miracle of life happens in us! It happens again every
single millisecond![13]

## 6. Intestinal health

'Death sits in the intestine,' said the doctors of Antiquity. Very early
on it was discovered that essentially all organic diseases develop in
the intestine. Early cultures with their very good knowledge of
medicine also researched this topic and gave us practical help for our
lives.[14] In Ayurvedic medicine this fact has been known for a long
time. Egyptian priests and the physicians of Ancient Greece and Rome
also gained knowledge of the subject. It is also known from the

information passed down from the advanced Mayan civilisations.

Our intestine is living. It is full of viruses and bacteria that absolutely belong there. What is fatal is that in our society we have managed to ruin our intestines through our lifestyle and 'prosperity' by swallowing and injecting chemicals from the pharmaceutical industry.

The results are particularly clear after medical treatment with antibiotics, antimycotics, cortisone preparations and other pharmaceuticals. In 2009, 40 million packs of antibiotics were prescribed in Germany. With an average of 30 tablets or capsules, from small packs for individuals to the large packets used in hospitals, this is equivalent to a yearly consumption of 1.2 billion tablets. This sum is prescribed by doctors in Germany alone.

For several years, certain doctors in Germany have been warning that we should be prescribing far fewer antibiotics. A runny nose or a cold, for example, can be easily cleared up with nasal rinsing and gargling with alkaline bath salts or salt water solution with thyme. Another very effective prophylactic is aronia berry juice. I was advised by a friend, who is a popular healer in his home town in Switzerland, that at the first signs of a cold I should make sure my kidneys and adrenal glands were given a great deal of warmth (with a kidney warmer or hot water bottle) and to treat my intestine with a zapper or healing crystal below the belly button for around 20 minutes. No antibiotics are required.

What does 'antibiotic' actually mean? It comes from the Greek 'anti' and

vaccinations. All of these substances contain heavy metals, for example mercury.

The main cause is amalgam which, for example, is used in fillings for teeth. Amalgam consists of:

58% mercury
16% tin
19% silver

15% copper and nickel, also known as high copper amalgam.

Heavy metals in the mouth affect the liver, kidneys and brain due to
salivation alone. These effects are increased by food which is too hot
or too acidic. This leads to gradual toxification with mild to severe
symptoms such as discomfort, kidney failure, nerve damage, brain
damage, a weakened immune system, inflammation, skin irritation
and psychological conditions such as depression.
We do not perceive this toxification directly. It develops within us over
decades.
However, all other diseases are also recognisable in our blood at
an early stage. Dark field microscopy allows diseases in the blood
to be recognised that have not yet made themselves apparent in
the body through complaints and pains.
In the last few years before my Parkinson's disease manifested
itself openly, from around 2000 onwards, I felt burning tears in
my eyes. This could be when I was reading, watch television or in
a meeting and began to happen more and more frequently. If I
drove for an extended period of time I often had to stop and let
someone else take over. I simply could not see anymore. Was
this overacidification? The signs pointed to uveitis, an
autoimmune disease. Around five years ago, before going blind,
my mother had also suffered constant pain due to similar acidic,
irritating tears that affected her retinas. No one could help her.
She was constantly being treated by different doctors and
optometrists. Of course I was scared that over time my disease
would take me down the same path as my mother.
Due to the dark field microscopy examinations, the treatment that
stemmed from them, the lifestyle I practice, and other things, these
symptoms have also disappeared completely.

People need to be considered as a whole. Everyone should practice this
themselves. Know yourself, love yourself and accept yourself! This
strong, unshakeable intention alone is often enough to influence the

over 40,000 pure memory cells in our organic hearts so positively that we can heal. The miracle of life happens in us! It happens again every single millisecond![13]

## 6. Intestinal health

'Death sits in the intestine,' said the doctors of Antiquity. Very early on it was discovered that essentially all organic diseases develop in the intestine. Early cultures with their very good knowledge of medicine also researched this topic and gave us practical help for our lives.[14] In Ayurvedic medicine this fact has been known for a long time. Egyptian priests and the physicians of Ancient Greece and Rome also gained knowledge of the subject. It is also known from the information passed down from the advanced Mayan civilisations.

Our intestine is living. It is full of viruses and bacteria that absolutely belong there. What is fatal is that in our society we have managed to ruin our intestines through our lifestyle and 'prosperity' by swallowing and injecting chemicals from the pharmaceutical industry.
The results are particularly clear after medical treatment with antibiotics, antimycotics, cortisone preparations and other pharmaceuticals. In 2009, 40 million packs of antibiotics were prescribed in Germany. With an average of 30 tablets or capsules, from small packs for individuals to the large packets used in hospitals, this is equivalent to a yearly consumption of 1.2 billion tablets. This sum is prescribed by doctors in Germany alone.
For several years, certain doctors in Germany have been warning that we should be prescribing far fewer antibiotics. A runny nose or a cold, for example, can be easily cleared up with nasal rinsing and gargling with alkaline bath salts or salt water solution with thyme. Another very effective prophylactic is aronia berry juice. I was advised by a friend, who is a popular healer in his home town in Switzerland, that at the first signs of a cold I should make sure my kidneys and adrenal glands were given a great deal of warmth (with a kidney warmer or

hot water bottle) and to treat my intestine with a zapper or healing crystal below the belly button for around 20 minutes. No antibiotics are required.

What does 'antibiotic' actually mean? It comes from the Greek 'anti' and 'bios', which literally translates to 'against life'. This is exactly what happens when we take antibiotics. All life in the intestine is destroyed. The consequence of this is that the intestine can no longer function properly; certain fungi and viruses can mutate and get into the blood through the intestine wall which has become holey or porous and cause even greater damage there.

Industrially produced meat that is sold for a low price in supermarkets comes from animals that have been loaded with vaccines (e.g. mercury, formaldehyde) and antibiotics during their short lives. Genetically modified soya and corn add to this. These substances remain in the meat after slaughtering of course. There are many people who are proud to eat these bargains. A lack of knowledge (and not wanting to know) lets them act this way.

I simply find it repulsive. These warnings now also apply to certain types of fish that come from fish farms. Here, like the animals mentioned above, the fish are given unnatural feed additives and medication, meaning they are no longer fit to eat.

For this reason, I always pay careful attention to the origins of any meat and fish that I buy. You should only eat fish that has been caught from the sea and other natural bodies of water. It is a legal obligation for producers of meat, fish and other food to state its origin. Please pay attention to this.

The condition of the intestine can be evaluated with dark field microscopy. Homeopathic methods to detoxify the body of heavy metals, viruses, bacteria and other things that make us ill fight such foreign substances. This can be done using Rizol, chlorella, and Froximun, for example. Black cumin, broad-leaved garlic and coriander are important components. The main causes of intestinal problems are poor nutrition, taking antibiotics and, above all, the mercury often found in amalgam fillings and a lack of exercise.[15]

Fortunately there are some responsible doctors who, after their patients have been treated with antibiotics that are genuinely required, ensure that their intestinal flora is restored. This is another important criterion by which to evaluate your doctor.
Therapies that use homeopathic preparations work in a completely different way. *Nothing* in the body or blood is killed. Harmful substances are simply removed. These gentle and effective methods can be used to successfully treat many diseases, including epidemic diseases.[16]


## 7. Rudolf Breuss' treatment

I will probably continue to use this method, which I found to be fantastic, to my benefit for the rest of my life. I did my first course of Breuss treatment over a period of 42 days in 2006. Since then I have been repeating it once a year for one to two weeks each time. I am incredibly enthusiastic about this simple, low-cost method, which has unbeatable results.
The treatment was developed by Rudolf Breuss (1899–1990), an Austrian practitioner of alternative medicine, for cancer patients.[17] Decades of observations and experience showed him that cancers and the substances which cause them live off solid food in our bodies.
Therefore, according to Breuss' conclusions, solid food should be avoided for a set period of time. And Rudolf Breuss healed thousands of patients with his vegetable juice course developed especially for this purpose.
Specifically, this means that in order to starve the harmful cells and remove them from the body no solid food is consumed for a period of 42 days. To ensure that patients do not starve Breuss developed his vegetable juice that contains all of the vitamins and minerals that the body needs. Today this juice is produced by the Swiss company Biotta

and its main ingredients are the juices from beetroot, celeriac, carrots, radishes and potatoes. During the first three weeks of the treatment I also took Breuss' kidney tea made of specific herbs to purify my kidneys. This tea is made of horsetail, nettles, knotgrass and St John's wort. I also took other teas, such as geranium tea, Epiloboum parviflorum tea and, last but not least, my beloved sage tea that I have been drinking on an empty stomach on a daily basis ever since. All the recipes, including one for a clear onion soup, can be found in Breuss' handbook *The Breuss Cancer Cure*. This book is a must for anyone who is in any way affected by cancer.
His book also contains advice for diseases such as angina, arteriosclerosis, biliary colic (very effective – I have tried it myself), rheumatism, trigeminal neuralgia and diabetes. It also provides information of Breuss' pain-free method of spinal adjustment.
'But,' I so often hear, 'I don't have cancer, what use is this cure to me?' Based on my experience, I advise people suffering from any form of disease to do Breuss' cancer cure and kidney purification treatments in order to thoroughly purify the body from the inside out. It is easier than you think not to eat anything solid for 42 days. If it had been necessary I would have been able to add a few more days on at the end.
Interestingly, during the treatment a bowel movement occurs between once a day and once every three days. Therefore, the body purifies itself and gently removes all harmful substances, all the things that make us ill, from the body. The treatment is low-cost as no food is required for its duration. You should make sure that your fridge is empty so that there are no temptations nearby. During the treatment, in addition to teas and good quality water, drinks made from vitamin-rich fresh juices, organic sauerkraut juice, celeriac juice and similar provide a nice amount of variety. Of course, after three weeks the body becomes a little weak, but a daily walk in the fresh air lasting at least an hour is essential. It clears the head. Easy office work can be easily completed.

Here the following tip is especially important: give up smoking beforehand, something which should be done in general but especially before the treatment, and which you should really not go back to afterwards.


8. Health in the environment and the home
A more apt heading would perhaps be 'Healing our sick environment', but then it would be difficult to know where to start...

First of all, the microwave that we often use but is not good for our health should disappear from the home. Research has shown that food heated in the microwave damages our health. The bioavailability of nutrients such as fats, proteins, carbohydrates, vitamins and minerals is dramatically reduced. After reheating food in general and especially in the microwave these substances can no longer be absorbed and processed by the body.
Up to 90 percent of the vital energy in all food that has been tested is lost. This leads to structural decay in all food, as well as overacidification and toxification in the body and, finally, cancer.[18] Microwaves do not just destroy the food heated in them but usually also harm people nearby.

Try the following test: place your mobile phone, switched on, in the microwave (do not turn the microwave on of course) and call your phone number from a different telephone. When your mobile phone rings this will show you that the microwaves can travel both in and out of the microwave. No further proof is required.[19]

We cannot fight the electro smog that comes from antennae and mobile phones, radar and electric devices, even cars, aeroplanes and trains. It is simply there. The flickering of fluorescent lights, although it is not visible to us, has a direct harmful effect on brain waves, as current EEGs (electroencephalography – a method of recording brainwaves) show.

The radio waves produced by mobile phones and cordless telephones in the home and office make is easier for the impurities circulating in the blood such as toxins, heavy metals and viruses to pass through the blood-brain barrier without a problem. Without these radio waves they would be rejected by the brain. Electro smog is often caused, for example, by frequently using cordless telephones, by mobile phones and by the constant radiation from microwaves that come from mobile phone masts. These can also damage our health. Mobile phones that are kept in a trouser pocket or attached to belts are known to be partly responsible for prostate and uterine cancer, for example.

Radiation from laptops balanced on the stomach or knees is just as dangerous. (The instructions for these devices even warn against these potential dangers!)

Reduce the electro smog wherever you can. It is not just mobile phones; cordless telephones, yes, even household ones with mobile docking stations, constantly emit harmful radiation even when they are not being used. If you do not need the Wi-Fi connection on your computer for any period of time then simply switch the Wi-Fi router off to avoid harmful radiation. Ask for advice at a specialist shop; solutions or at least initial steps towards solutions have been developed. Consumers only have to ask persistently to defend their health. Televisions must be removed from the bedroom. Ideally you should use a special switch (mains disconnector) to turn off all electricity overnight. Radio alarm clocks and lamps with transformers (halogen lamps, lamps with dimmers) emit harmful radiation even when switched off. An electrician can advise you on the easiest method to counteract this.

And what about that new car? It takes two years for all of the harmful substances in the paint, glue, upholstery, etc. to evaporate. Does this mean that a used car is healthier?

Renovation work in the home is also a problem. New floors and wall panels, paint and glue contaminate the air. Sometimes it cannot be tolerated.

Water is also of key significance. We are told that tap water is the most well controlled thing that we consume. Unfortunately, however, in recent years the maximum permitted values have become higher and higher, meaning that the quality has worsened compared to 30 years ago. The additives prescribed by the government alone, such as chlorine, fluoride and iodine, are essentially disguised toxins. They have a particularly strong effect in swimming pools. On top of this there are the contaminants that depend of the time of year and the location, such as nitrates that come from fertilisers.

The fact is that the government has increased the maximum values tenfold over the past 20 years to suit these contaminants. An independent water quality inspector at a local swimming pool recently brashly told me that this was the price of civilisation.

Chlorinated water in swimming pools is absorbed in particularly high quantities by children aged two and under. Problems with the bronchi can occur. Coupled with the generous asthma inhaler treatment from the doctor, this ensures asthma will develop in the future. Could this be wrong? After all, the inhalers have nice pictures of bears on them these days!

It would be more sensible to recommend that parents avoid taking their children swimming in chlorinated water during the first two years of their lives. The May 2010 issue of *Apotheken Umschau* magazine mentions a study by the University of Leuven in Belgium which analysed data on 450 children, most of whom were under two years of age. The researchers discovered a high frequency of inflammation in the fine branches of the bronchi; this in turn increases the risk of developing asthma and allergies.[20]

Tap water and mineral water that is contaminated by uranium presents a particular danger. Putting 'safe for babies' on the bottle is often just an advertising trick. Check http://www.foodwatch.org/en/ for current information. Uranium, heavy metals, medication residue

and phosphate fertiliser affect the purity of all types of water in Germany. The government currently considers a maximum amount of 2 µg (microgrammes) per litre of water to be acceptable. However, the values measured in tap water across Germany range from 10 to 20µg per litre of water. Microfilters can be used to reduce these high amounts. Only the water companies are against this.
The German Federal Institute for Risk Assessment (yes, this really exists) requires companies to inform consumers of the uranium content on their packaging. According to findings by the German Federal Office of Consumer Protection and Food Safety, the maximum values should be increased to 10µg per litre of water due to the increased quantities. These increased quantities harm the kidney, brain and bones. The uranium content of the water that is used can even be identified in breast milk.

Smog in cities and tunnels, exhaust fumes, dust particles, minute pieces of tyres, asbestos from brake linings and fan belts, yes, even from washing machines and dryers, cause us harm. Even in aeroplanes we are exposed to a great deal of harmful things during take-off and landing. Kerosene from the air-conditioning unavoidably gets inside the cabin. And what happens during the flight? According to a television report in *plusminus* (ARD), during the flight the air in an aeroplane can be contaminated by TCP that is mixed into the engine oil.
31 swab samples taken from the cabins of aeroplanes belonging to different airlines tested 'positive' in 28 cases, with up to 154.9µg on 2cm². The permitted value is 0.00µg. This harmful TCP gets directly from the engine into the cabin, unfiltered, via what is known as bleed air. Air stewards suffer from this and often become ill.[21]

Smokers have to be addressed here too of course. It has been scientifically proven that the air breathed in from a cigarette is contaminated by over 600 different toxic, harmful substances. Substances such as hydrogen cyanide, arsenic, mercury, ammonia,

acetone and many more should really be something to think about.
They are life-threatening for both active and passive smokers.[22]

Genetic modification is an important topic for our environment;
manipulated life is playing an ever larger role. Genetic modification is
much more than just modified corn. Animals are manipulated, animal
feed is manipulated, trees, vegetables and fruit are manipulated.
Umweltinstitut München e. V. (www.umweltinstitut.org)  provides
explanations and has information brochures for all those who are
interested. Do we really want to eat pharmacological plants and
pharmacological animals? The terminator technology used by the
leading companies goes so far that the plants no longer produce
viable seeds. This means the manipulated seeds always have to be
bought from these companies at excessively high prices. This is called
profit optimisation in the 21$^{st}$ century... In certain areas in Africa it has
already got to the stage that farmers and their families starve
because they can no longer make enough money to buy genetically
modified corn seeds. Their soil is barren due to the much praised
artificial fertilisers. The people become ill.[23]
Alternative cultivation methods have been demonstrating for a long
time that returning to conventional methods and traditional varieties is
much more beneficial to our health. 70 percent of all farmers and
consumers in Europe are against genetically modified food.
Why are potatoes equipped with venom genes from scorpions,
strawberries with frost-protection genes from arctic fish or lettuces
with rat genes? Do we really want to eat genetically modified plants
which, at the same time, produce vaccines, antibodies or even
hormones? Genetic modification in animals is unacceptable, and not
just for ethical reasons. Pathological changes in the internal organs,
stomach ulcers, arthritis, kidney problems and skin diseases in
transgenetic pigs, and deformed bodies, heads and tumours in fish
send a very clear message.[24]

The ecological risks of transgenetic plants are made clear by the direct damage to flora and fauna. Cross-breeding genetically modified crop plants will in all likelihood cause wild plants (including those used in natural medicine) to die out due to transgenetic plants established themselves in the environment. The consequence of this is a change in the use of land due to increased use of pesticides and monoculture. Beekeeping will die out, as has already happened in certain countries. There are more and more indications that the concept of the so-called co-existence of genetically modified crops and conventional and organic agriculture is a lie. Genetically modified crops ensure that the companies that produce the seeds and pesticides can sell them as a two-in-one product. Other companies and the 'healthcare' industry then make large profits from the people who are made sick.[25]


## 9. Healing stone therapy

Healing stones are directly related to the minerals in the human body. The following stones have proven to be very helpful for my Parkinson's disease:

Chalcedony*
Gold-sheen obsidian
Fluorite**
Green tourmaline
Red-brown jasper, sanded into an olive shape*
Malachite
Mookaite*
Rhyolite
Schalenblende*
Silicon
Emerald*[26]
Star sapphire
Sodalite**

*      I have used these stones on my body and sometimes still do.
**      I use these stones in my 'healing stone water' along with quartz, rose quartz, amethyst, apatite and citrine.

The stones that are not marked by stars were good
recommendations that I have not tested on myself.
A specialist is required here. They can test the stones out on an
individual basis.
I have had particularly good experiences with emerald, citrine,
mookaite, jasper and chalcedony.

I wore the cream-coloured mookaite on a pendant throughout the day.
It became very warm and can sometimes feel uncomfortable. If this is
the case you should start by only wearing it for an hour at a time.
With the emeralds, in the early stages of my Parkinson's disease I
used surgical tape to tape an emerald crystal from Columbia to my
head in the area where I was experiencing the most problems. Here I
felt the vibrations immediately. During the night I slept with simple
polished emeralds from India (similar to worry stones) on my pillow.
The jasper was used to strengthen my sense of smell that I lost due
to Parkinson's disease. I placed an olive-shaped piece of jasper in one
nostril and then the other for an hour at a time (when I was watching
television, for example).
After three to five months, the effect that the vibrations of all of these
crystals had on me was that finally my ears started producing ear
wax again and when I woke up in the morning I had sleep in my eyes
once more. I was very happy about this because these natural
occurrences had been absent for years.
Today I still wear a chalcedony bracelet on my wrist to support my
concentration and mental agility. At the same time, thanks to its
effect on organs such as the liver and gallbladder, the chalcedony
also helps prevent overacidification.
*Tip:* Never work at a laptop or computer while wearing healing stone
bracelets, rings or pendants. The vibrations of the stones can affect
them so much that they cause errors and faults, particularly with the
integrated mouse function on laptops.
A specialist can determine the stone that corresponds to your
astrological sign. The chapter on water crystals explains which healing

stones can be placed in water to produce energised water for drinking and cooking.

Scientists are now able to visualise and document the vibrations of healing stones and crystals through photon photography. Bioresonance measurements can also identify the vibrations of healing stones and crystals very exactly (in nanometres). And, finally, anyone who is familiar with how to use a pendulum can measure the energy of healing stones and crystals in Bovis units.[27]

## 10. Physiotherapy

It is essential for Parkinson's sufferers to find a suitable physiotherapist. This is not always easy. The only way is to try and observe. Before treatment, ask specifically whether there is a specialist for Parkinson's disease available. (You may also want to seek information from your health insurance provider; when retraining people as massage therapists they often used to say things like 'You're a baker? Well then you can knead well.')

It is no use if the practice simply has a reputation for offering outstanding massages or other therapies. What you need is a therapist with specialist training for Parkinson's disease. Such therapists will choose targeted exercises which focus on coordination between the body and mind in order to improve concentration. My best experiences were with therapists who came from clinics for stroke, Parkinson's and Alzheimer's patients. The therapist's touch begins in the heart. The way of judging a good therapist is the effect of their touch. To touch the body and in doing so touch the soul – this should be the foundation of a therapist's work. A patient's external appearance reflects their soul and their uniqueness.

The soul is exposed completely. At this point at the very latest, you will feel the benefits of the perceptive abilities of a good therapist whose intuition allows them to touch the soul as much as the body. The first touch, the first time a hand strokes my back, tells me whether I as a patient have been accepted, with body, mind and soul.

The hands of a well-trained, sensitive therapist activate more powers in me than any word. This touch can even help and provide comfort for my spiritual pain.

In my discussions with sufferers I have discovered that people often wait with longing for their appointments. The value of a treatment lies in the touch and in the discussion as a whole. Good physiotherapy is much more than just a good massage. Please also try at home. Have the exercises explained in detail. The success of this treatment could be increased significantly if all patients continued it at home on a daily basis.

Occupational therapy: This focuses first and foremost on the fine motor skills of the hands and facial gestures. Everything that is required for daily life is practiced; even simple things such as eating and getting dressed must sometimes be relearnt. As some patients' handwriting becomes illegible, writing exercises are also part of good occupational therapy. Always make sure all exercises are demonstrated and explained in detail. You should also practice them yourself several times a day at home. Do not be afraid to ask!

A friend of mine who looks after children with ADD and ADHD showed me another very helpful exercise that he does with the children for around 10 minutes before school starts, where you draw the number eight on its side as a concentration exercise.

I have discovered that this is also a good exercise for me as a Parkinson's patient, and is also useful in connection with the writing exercises. You will find that after a few days, handwriting that was scrawled becomes fluid again. With practice the loops in the number eight also become more even. This is a simple but highly efficient method of training both halves of the brain. All of these exercises should be carried out in a playful manner.

I recommend that Parkinson's sufferers use a soft trampoline to train their brains' coordination skills and their sense of balance. The power plate that is used by physiotherapists is also sufficient for targeted balance exercises.

Feldenkrais therapy: This therapy is very successful when it comes to coordinating brain function and the body. Moshé Feldenkrais began his research and experiments in neuropsychology and behavioural psychology around 1940. He later taught at universities in North America, at the Sorbonne in France, in Israel and in England. His most famous students included Ben Gurion, Yehudi Menuhin, Peter Brooke and Franz Wurm from Zürich, who leads the Feldenkrais Institute there.[28]

According to Moshé Feldenkrais the body is the guardian of truth. Every cell is addressed. A therapeutic relationship is still a relationship. New ways of understanding the body and soul are developed.

From my own experience I can say that these exercises which use very small, fine movements activate the brain in a way that is almost imperceptible but all the more sustainable for it. The body is supported intensively and relaxed at the same with special exercises and small movements. I recommend one-on-one therapy sessions as they ensure the best possible success through the interaction between the teacher and the student (patient). I was very fortunate to have one of the best Feldenkrais guides from 1999 to 2005. I have never met a more helpful, selfless therapist.

Speech therapy: The typical swallowing problems and unclear speech are a clear sign that the help of a speech therapist is required. Through simple breathing exercises the oxygen supply to the voice which is gradually becoming hoarse and quiet is improved. Pronunciation is practiced. The articulation, rhythm and volume of speech are improved. First and foremost you should practice reading aloud. Read more and more loudly over time. This is very important in this context.

Yoga exercises are an everyday part of my life. They should be compulsory for all Parkinson's sufferers. Yoga improves concentration and relaxation, and promotes an understanding of one's own body and love for the body and its potential.[29]

Learning to accept yourself as you are, to recognise small improvements and feel child-like, honest happiness; this is how I enjoy my hour of yoga every week – without false ambition, I simply let things happen.

Yoga is good for people who can also sense the spiritual background. This enriches the experience as it means that the exercises are put into practice not just physically but also psychologically. For people who are more pragmatically minded, yoga is a sequence of wonderful physical actions that always follow on logically from one another and complement each other. Yoga helps. If I am ever unable to go to my yoga class I have an exercise CD that I can use at home and always take with me when I go away.

Dorn-Breuss therapy: This therapy is based on two different therapies. I have already mentioned the Austrian practitioner of alternative medicine Rudolf Breuss and his diverse treatment methods.[30]

The special massage method developed by Rudolf Breuss is based on the experience that there are usually no damaged disks. Pain is usually caused by discs being out of place, which in turn leads to a narrowing of the vertebral foramina and can stimulate or even trap the nerves there. Breuss' basic idea was that the discs, which act as shock absorbers, often contain too little liquid (which is usually seen as wear).

A disc can be thought of as a sponge. During the day this sponge is squashed between the vertebrae and put under pressure until it is only a few millimetres thick. If we have drunk enough during the day, the disc can absorb liquid again overnight so that it can function as the perfect shock absorber again the next day. This is why we are a little taller in the morning than in the evening.

The Dorn method developed by Dieter Dorn considers the spine, hips and pelvis as a whole. His method, which was developed largely on the basis of rural home remedies, has not just made life more bearable for many patients but actually relieved them of their pain entirely.[31]

Unlike chiropractic treatment, the Dorn method makes corrections by pressing a finger gently on the spinous process or the transverse process of the incorrectly placed vertebra. The patient stands or sits for the treatment and aids the therapy through their own small movements. The only tools used in the treatment are the therapist's hands which see the spine as the 'soul of the body'.

A complementary method is the Breuss-Dorn-Fleig method.[32] As a student of Rudolf Breuss and Dieter Dorn, Harald Fleig learnt their methods and the ways in which they could help people. He applied this knowledge effectively himself and is now one of the most highly regarded trainers in this area.

Dental reflexology: The charts for foot reflexology are now well known internationally; they present a complicated picture of the structures, organs and meridians. Dental reflexology (Latin: dens = tooth; reflex = the body's response to a stimulus), however, is a method of diagnosing and treating diseased teeth and their interference fields in relation to physical diseases. Sources of disease and interference fields are cases of chronic inflammation which are encapsulated in the body. We are familiar with this in the tonsils, sinuses and appendix. Yet up to 80 percent of sources and interference fields are in the teeth.[33] They may be cavities, the remains of roots, dead teeth, teeth that have had root canal treatment, inflammation of the gums or unsuccessful orthodontic treatment, for example. The canines are responsible for shoulder pain, migraines, lymphatic congestion, gallbladder problems, flatulence, urogenital inflammation, and endocarditis, but also for psychological problems. In dental reflexology the relationships in the body become clearer. For example, the nervous tissue of the third/fourth cervical vertebra is responsible for the shoulder reflex.

However, it also shows whether the top right canine or another tooth is affected. Treatments are carried out with a reflex laser that is used on the wall of the bone or the dental tissue from a distance of just 635 nm.

All problems with the pelvis, such as pelvis obliquity or even a barely noticeable change in the position of the pelvis, caused by the wing of the ilium, change the spine; this changes the situation in the jaw and changes the bite completely.

A misaligned jaw, often caused by pelvis obliquity, can then lead to completely different problems, such as facial pain, earache, migrating toothache, ringing in the ears, grinding teeth, lymphatic congestion, sinus problems, nerve and brain damage, inflammation, skin irritation, weakened immune defence and many more. During treatment a specialist dentist will often work together with a physiotherapist who is experienced in reflexology.


## 11. Meridian therapy

The body's energy channels are called meridians, a term that comes from traditional Chinese medicine (TCM). In these channels flows the chi, the Chinese term for life force energy. This life force energy flows through our bodies in a way that can be likened to a river system flowing across a map.

The meridians form a very complex system. There are 12 main meridians that connect all of the internal organs, and 8 known as extraordinary meridians. The acupressure and acupuncture points through which the chi can be manipulated to treat disease can be found along the meridians.

This ancient knowledge has now been accepted by some enlightened doctors who have recognised the potential of natural medicine and make it available to their patients. The bioenergy specialist Dr Albrecht Hempel, a researcher at the department of orthopaedics at the hospital in Neustadt[34] and at Friedrich Schiller University Jena[35], has carried out clinical studies and double-blind studies which

demonstrate the effectiveness of acupuncture.
For a long time, life force energy, the chi and the meridians were almost mythical terms that were dismissed as esoteric beliefs. However, now it is possible to make the meridian channels and the flow of life force energy visible in the form of electromagnetic impulses, energy fields and coloured interference using photon photography. I have been using this knowledge of the meridians on an almost daily basis for years (see part I, Meridian seminar). It is indispensable, especially for the tremor and the interaction of the nerves and brain.

In the beginning my daily practical exercises were as follows: for the tremor on the right I found the meridian pressure point on the back left edge of the skull around the height of the earlobe. Of course, the position varies slightly from person to person, but we can all feel the point, particularly as this area usually hurts a little. I then pressed and massaged this point for three minutes; over the following days I increased this to ten minutes.
If it hurt too much I only pressed lightly to start with. Everyone develops their own feel for this. The important thing is to do it regularly – at least once a day, up to three times in the beginning. With time the tremor will improve considerably.
The second, equally important meridian point for Parkinson's sufferers is the central nervous system's point which is found in the middle of the skull. To find it you will initially need a second person to help you. Looking at the head from above, a line should be imagined from the middle of one ear to the middle of the other ear, and a line from the nasal bone over the head and down to the spine. At the point where these two lines cross a small hollow can be felt. This is the central nervous system's meridian point which should be stimulated. This is slightly difficult in the beginning but with practice you will be able to find the point yourself because you will be able to feel it. In the meridian course that I took we were given a specially designed stick for this exercise by a Mr Thai from Lucerne.[36] This stimulation activates the nervous system very effectively – without

medication, without side effects and without toxins.

Today the latter exercise is part of my daily ritual. However, I now use neither the stick nor my hands but simply concentrate on this point during my meditation. This is enough. The effect is the same.
However, it requires you to involve the universe and its powerful energies.
For this reason, I ask for help in all of my plans. Regardless of whether I want to supply myself with energy to activate my powers of self-healing or whether I want to support other people. Of course, this works in the same way for most other diseases.
Working with the meridian points helps greatly here.
There are of course a whole range of other meridian points that are significant for Parkinson's sufferers. As there are different symptoms there are also different types of treatment. I therefore recommend that you discuss these therapies individually with a therapist; this chapter is simply intended to highlight their potential.


## 12. Craniosacral therapy

As I explained in the first part of this book, this is a special form of therapy that releases blockages and tensions in the body. The causes of such problems may include falls, sitting in the wrong position or shock. The lymph nodes are also simulated considerably.

Craniosacral therapy (Latin: cranium = skull; sacrum = the bone at the base of the spine) is based on ancient Native American healing practices and has recently begun to be taught at schools for alternative practitioners in Germany.
Dr Andrew Taylor Still, the son of a priest and doctor who began studying to become a doctor like his father in Kansas in 1853, is considered the founder of this therapy. He qualified as a doctor in 1861 and worked as a military doctor during the American Civil war until 1864. After four of his five children died very young from

meningitis and pneumonia, he turned away from the church and the established medical institutions and began searching for new methods of healing. He studied bone setting, a form of medicine practiced by the Shawnee Native Americans, and also followed the developments being made in medicine in Europe and America with particular interest.
The concept of a healing magnetism, which had already been used in mesmerism, refers to the circulation of a universal fluid. Today we know that what is meant here is the cerebrospinal fluid that is also closely linked to the brain. Andrew Taylor Still discovered that anatomical disruptions led to blockages in the blood and the lymph system or could block the nerves. He was publically criticised for this by those in conventional medicine. Yet he had introduced the term osteopathy (Greek: osteon = bones; Greek: pathie = suffering) for this type of treatment in 1874. Still's new practice in Missouri had already had great success with this method of therapy back in 1851. In 1892, he founded the American School of Osteopathy. Cranial osteopathy was developed at the beginning of the 19th century by Dr William Garner Sutherland, a former student of Dr Still's, on the basis of his work in osteopathy.
Another of Still's students was Dr Daniel David Palmer who became famous as the founder of modern chiropractic. Craniosacral therapy in its current form was researched further by one of William Sutherland's students and expanded with many practical suggestions that can be used on a day-to-day basis. Today Dr John Upledger is one of the most well-known advocates of craniosacral therapy.[37]

Together with the cerebral membrane and the meninges, the two fixed points of this therapy – the skull (cranium) and sacrum – form a unit in which the cerebrospinal fluid pulses rhythmically. What is crucial here is to feel the movements of the skull seams of the 26 skulls bones, as well as the expansion and contraction of the brain, which is surrounded by the fluid. These impulses in the cerebral membrane and meninges continue from the brain through the vertebral canal down to the sacrum.

Dr Sutherland discovered that this rhythm can be compared to the heartbeat; it is a distinct, unique power in our bodies. Sutherland called this the 'breath of life'. It expresses itself throughout the body and can be compared to the breathing of the lungs (the secondary respiration) and to the breathing of the tissues of the central nervous system. These three levels of breathing regulate all of the body's functions.

The therapeutic effect of craniosacral therapy accelerates and supports the healing process in a wide range of diseases. I recommend craniosacral therapy for all Parkinson's sufferers. The treatments last around an hour and are carried out lying down. My experiences with this therapy have been very good and I still have a treatment session once a month with therapists who I find very gifted and selfless. I am sure you will be able to find a therapist nearby by looking online. [38]


## 13. Singing bowl therapy (based on my intuition)

Singing bowls have been used for healing in Tibet for thousands of years with great and small success. The patient feels the vibrations of the singing bowl in their body and experiences profound centring and harmonisation. The powers of self-healing are activated. You hear not just with your ears but, in a way, with your whole body.

The sounds create calm but also movement and healing. Singing bowl therapy has a very calming effect on patients. The vibrations of the singing bowls bring about a state of deep calm in the brain which is very pleasant for Parkinson's sufferers.

Unfortunately, there are currently only a small number of really good therapists. As this treatment is used by some people for spa treatments its spiritual background is often ignored.

Disease always comes hand in hand with disharmony in the body. Working with singing bowls can help to release blocked energies through harmonic vibrations. This is similar to the way that a pebble creates ripples in water. The lymph nodes benefit from these vibrations immediately; the effect is truly astounding.

*Before continuing, please note the following:* The mallet used to strike the singing bowl must have a felt head. The standard wooden mallet is not suitable for this exercise.

My morning exercise is as follows: After taking a shower I lie down in a relaxed position on the bed with the mallet next to me ready to be picked up. Then I breathe in an out consciously at least three times, with my stomach expanding greatly as I breathe in and with my stomach muscles pulling in as far as possible as I breathe out. Each breath in and out should last three to four seconds. After this conscious breathing exercise I return to breaking normally. Next I place the singing bowl on my rib cage by the thymus and strike the bowl slowly and gently three times. After each strike I wait for the vibrations to stop.

In my head I say the following after each strike:

*I love my God.*

*I love my soul.*

*I love my body.*

Then I place the singing bowl on my upper stomach, strike it three more times, saying each time in my head:

*I love my stomach organs.*

*I love my blood.*

*I love my cells.*

If you have problems with a specific stomach organ you should also name the organ and place the singing bowl over it. Next I place the singing bowl on my lower stomach and say again in my head:

*I love my stomach organs.*

*I love my lymph nodes.*

*I love my cells.*

Then I place the singing bowl on my left thigh, strike it slowly three more times and say:

*I love my left leg.*

Then I place the singing bowl on the knee and say my affirmation again. Then I place it on my right thigh. Next comes the right knee and then the feet. As it is not possible to reach the feet without help you need to bend your knees and pull them towards yourself. After a little time you should raise your feet by around 20cm to strengthen the stomach muscles. While doing this I lift my head so that I can easily reach the singing bowl with by back stretched into a rounded position. My head is then around the level of my knees.

Parkinson's sufferers often lose feeling in their feet. I did this exercise once a day for two years before I was finally able to feel the vibration of the singing bowl. Therefore, I ask you to please be patient with yourself.
If I have time I combine the singing bowl therapy with a few other therapeutic exercises. My legs are already bent and raised slightly. I then wrap my arms around them and carefully turn them right and left. While doing this I turn my head in the opposite direction. This strengthens the spine. You should carry out this exercise carefully to start with. Beginning with 3 to 5 turns in each direction, you should later increase this to 30 to 50.

In another important exercise I make sure my feet are flat with my knees still bent and my bottom is raised as far as possible (bridge). As I do so, with all my concentration, I lift my left and right leg a few centimetres in turn and then put it back down again. I know that for the first few months this is very difficult for Parkinson's sufferers. To strengthen the abdominal wall – a weak abdominal wall is responsible for most back problems – I lie on my back and make a cycling motion with my legs. To start with you can do this just 5 to 10 times but later you can increase it to 70 to 80.

I ensure I am relaxed and take my time with all of these exercises. Then I take my left hand and place the singing bowl underneath it on the wrist and carpal tunnel (especially important for carpal tunnel

syndrome). I strike it slowly and carefully three more times, wait for the vibrations and say in my head:
*I love my left hand.*
You should take your time and enjoy the vibrations until they come to an end after each strike. Next is the left elbow, which is treated in the same way. I bend my arm a little to secure the bowl. In my head I say:
*I love my left arm.*
Then I do the same on the right. I relax for a moment, stretch my legs, my big toes touching. I place the singing bowl back on my rib cage. I strike it three more times, harder this time, at steady intervals one after the other, while saying in my head:
*I love my thymus.*
*I love my spine.*
*I love my cells.*
Here you should feel the vibrations from the ribs to the spine. It takes a while before the whole body shows the desired responses. Therefore, please be patient with yourself.
After a short pause I lay my head on its right side and carefully place the singing bowl on the left side. I strike it very lightly and quietly three more times and particularly enjoy the sound and the vibration. The position of the singing bowl hear stimulates the lymph nodes in the inner ear that regulate balance. I say in my head each time:
*I love the left side of my brain.*
Now I remove the singing bowl, turn my head back to the middle, take three deep breaths and turn my head onto its left side. Once again I strike to bowl very lightly quietly and say in my head:
*I love the right side of my brain.*
Finally, as the highlight of the singing bowl therapy, I turn my head back to the middle, place the singing bowl carefully on my forehead and say:
*I love my God.*
*I love my soul.*
*I love all of my cells.*

Then I remove the bowl and allow the sensations that I have felt to linger for a few minutes. (By the way, this is not about hearing the sounds but feeling the vibrations.)
The vibrations of the singing bowl calm us at the cell level and can therefore activate profound healing effects. I feel as if I have been reborn. What a wonderful day! Try it for yourself. It is a fantastic start to a new day.


## 14. Consciousness therapy with Bach flower remedies

Dr Edward Bach (1886–1936) discovered the effect of Bach flowers in the 1920s and developed a therapy for all diseases that reacts to certain states of consciousness.[39] These states are, for example, fear, envy, jealously, loneliness, a need for recognition, guilt and feelings of shock.
Edward Bach practiced as a doctor, researchers and bacteriologist in London. While he was there he began working with the flower concentrations that he had developed, but it was not until he retired to Mount Vernon in Oxfordshire that he completed his research. Today the well-known Bach Centre that he established is located there. It still produces the mother tinctures that he developed and that are diluted and put into smaller bottles. They often still use plants from the locations that Dr Bach found in his time. Bach flower therapy teaches how to deal with negative states of mind. The long-term therapy aims to bring harmony to the soul and to allow the personality to develop and stabilise as much as possible. The Bach flower remedies are not suitable for organic diseases but are very helpful for emotional problems, such as insecurity, oversensitivity, apathy, despondency, despair and similar emotions.
As Parkinson's disease is partly a psychological disease, the suitable Bach flower remedies can strengthen the patient's character which will help them to overcome the disease.
Dr Jentschura recommends the following: gorse, mustard, olive, sweet chestnut and rockwater.[40] In the beginning, Bach rescue

remedies were able to help me in certain difficult situations, such as during treatment, doctor's appointments, examinations such as MRI scans, examinations using radioactive contrast substances, and PET examinations.

The remedies are made of a mixture of 5 flower essences:
1. Cherry plum
2. Clematis
3. Impatiens
4. Rock rose
5. Star of Bethlehem

The selection from the Bach flower remedies, of which there are over 40, should be done by a specialist. Finding the right concentration may seem easy but I recommend that you seek expert advice, especially before taking them for the first time. It is not as easy as it is sometimes made out to be. Why not?

Because we would need to be able to assess and recognise ourselves properly. However, our partners, siblings, children and friends sometimes know us better than we know ourselves. Today I use my pendulum to determine the right concentration for me. The pharmacy is then happy to make the mixture.
*Tip:* Make sure that you inform the pharmacist if the remedy is intended for someone who must not consume alcohol, even in small amounts. If this is the case they will use cider vinegar as the carrier substance instead of alcohol, which is normally used.


## 15. Heavy metal detoxification

Here it is important to keep the following in mind: the journey is the destination. Because we are not ill, we are poisoned! Under state supervision, if we do not resist, we are damaged by the 'blessings' of the pharmaceutical and food industries. Most things you can get at the

supermarket are not really good for you!
Heavy metals mainly get into the body from dental amalgam.
Around 30 tonnes of mercury amalgam are currently processed in the USA every year. Amalgam is now banned in Sweden, Japan and Russia.
In Germany, however, it is still widely used in fillings, even though the first publications on the dangers of amalgam by Professor A. Stock appeared back in 1926 (it is thought that he had written up to 50 papers and publications by the end of his lifetime).[41]
Now that, in addition to formaldehyde, other substances such as mercury are used in vaccines (thiomersal), one in 150 children in the USA are autistic. As many as one in ten children show autistic tendencies such as problems reading and writing, but also other abnormal symptoms such as Rett syndrome or Asperger's syndrome.[42]

Many studies have shown that the heavy metals that have entered the blood through the camouflaged fungi in the intestine accumulate in the brain. This results in Alzheimer's disease, Parkinson's disease, multiple sclerosis and hyper activity, but also chronic tiredness and many other disorders. It can also cause problems sleeping.
Another symptom of toxification of the blood is that, with increased age, the mucosa dry out, which can lead to sinusitis and increased susceptibility to colds, flatulence and many other problems.
Furthermore, cravings for sweet things increase because the mutated fungi in the blood and brain urgently need this source of nutrition, which can in turn lead to severe additional overacidification. It is the same cycle over and over again.
Metals can also enter the body in adults through tattoos (iron oxide) or piercings (metal intolerance), permanent make up and tobacco consumption, but also through certain contaminated types of fish such as tuna, salmon and mackerel. Substances such as wood protector, weed killer, pesticides and insecticides all contain heavy metals that we end up consuming on a day-to-day basis through our food.

Metal toxification is then increased by aluminium packaging. Even aluminium saucepans and foil can lead to microfine particles entering the body, harming the nervous system and brain. Nanoparticles which are used as anti-caking agents are also often made from aluminium.[43, 44] All of these kinds of items should therefore be avoided.

Lead piping in old buildings increases the intake of heavy metals. Almost all people who live in industrialised European countries have increased levels of lead in their bodies which, in combination with the mercury mentioned above, leads to toxins being increased by a factor of ten.[45] Heavy metals can also enter the bloodstream in the form of palladium (the low-quality gold-coloured substance, slightly lighter than normal gold, that is used in fillings). A chemical compound of mercury amalgam and palladium increases the toxicity of mercury once again by a factor of ten. In such cases, a specialist should carry out dental restoration.[46]

The heavy metals enter into symbiosis with the intestinal fungi and enter the bloodstream through the intestine. From there they accumulate to a certain extent in the brain.

From my own experience, I know that an alternative practitioner can carry out a special heavy metal detoxification of the blood using natural homeopathic methods, but only after the fungi in the blood have been successfully removed.

The blood values can be diagnosed simply and quickly using dark field microscopy followed by radionic testing. Based on experience, detoxification is required in most cases. Heavy metals from amalgam, toxins, vaccines and food that have already begun to accumulate in tissue and form tumours in which harmful substances become stored are harder to remove.

One of the surest ways that I have found of removing cadmium, mercury and similar substances from the body has been chlorella algae products, sometimes together with Froximun products or with coriander and/or wild garlic tinctures, etc. Your alternative practitioner or doctor should decide on the course of treatment.[47]

## 16. Meditation

Every disease is a spiritual act, as every disease fulfils a spiritual task
in us. Trust yourself and the possibilities of healing that can happen
through trust and spirituality. There are many things in our lives that
we do not understand at first. Consciously place them in God's hands,
or whatever you wish to call God, and soon the understanding of
these rich possibilities of healing will enrich your life.
To trust yourself again is a wonderful experience.

Yet we do not know the way that is set out for us. We do not know
why we get this or that disease. No one knows.
Do you believe there is a form of guidance and fate in your life? If
you do then it is simple. If you firmly and resolutely believe in being
healed of a disease then it will happen. This is the practical
implementation of Matthew's words, 'If you believe, you will receive
whatever you ask for in prayer' (Matthew 21:22). This is how I feel
too. Of course, this does not mean that I immediately became
healthy again after asking. I am sure that my cells receive
information on how to heal more easily through my firm belief in
fulfilment. The healing process has been activated.
However, this is not enough to make you healthy again. I know some
Parkinson's sufferers who live in a state of expectation that this will
happen exactly according to these words. They pray and ask but still
do not become healthy again. Yet they reject all other forms of help
and advice.
How can that be? I believe that I can learn to connect the words of
the scripture to the little things that happen throughout my day.
Perhaps it is simply a pointer from a news programme or a telephone
call where I hear about a book that can help me further with my
experiences of the disease.
My spiritual guidance allows this information to come to me as if by

'coincidence'. I have prayed and prayed that I will become healthy again. I have endeavoured to understand the pointers that I receive, to accept them and put them into practice for myself.

I believe that this is the inner attitude for such as healing process. Accept everything with thanks! Because, if the miracle were to happen and you were to instantly become healthy again, you would continue with your previous lifestyle. Based on what I have learnt, I believe that this is why miracles do not happen in the way that some people imagine. The miracle happens very gradually once the spirit has understood why this healing is happening within me.

In my case, this is perhaps so that I can write this book and set up a self-help organisation to help people with the most diverse questions. Perhaps! I do not know. It is simply my experience of my disease and, now, my whole life.

Nowadays many people find it difficult to believe in God in the way that we have come to know or been presented with Him in our religious communities. Yet the awareness that there must be something more is there. And there is something.

I am convinced that it is the big energies of our universe that are readily available to everyone. It is not important whether we are Christians, Muslims, Buddhists, Jews or followers of any other beliefs, or even if we do not believe at all. What is important is simply that **HE** is there, **HE** loves us, **HE** heals us.

We do not need anything more. If we are supposed to be healed it will happen. This is how people healed other people thousands of years ago. They learnt a way of using the universe's endless energy for everyone – people, animals and plants. Anyone can recognise diseases and compensate for them with the universe's energy. Disease is a lack of energy or vibrations.

Only love and acceptance of nature, which is magnificent, can help us to understand. We can achieve this through meditation with deep relaxation.

Self-healing of our bodies happens through the power of thoughts in meditation.

I do not go a day without meditation in the morning and in the evening. I simply take a few minutes to immerse myself in spiritual and physical calm. By doing this I support the process of regeneration in my body and my health.

Many of us will remember saying our morning and evening prayers as children. Then most of us stopped saying them at some point. We prayed to the almighty God of our religion that our parents chose for us.

Today we know that God is not an old man with a long beard. But he exists. In space, in the universe, the almighty God is everywhere with his unbelievably energetic power. With a little practice we can all feel this. These are the moments, when we are alone with ourselves and our God or his spiritual guidance, when we can speak and ask urgently for help to heal and guidance to become healthy again. And also to give thanks, when we have received what we have prayed for.

If you do not believe in God, I recommend that you see this meditation simply as a quiet phase. Picture a pleasant scene, such as a beautiful landscape or clouds. Now breathe deeply in and out and try to think of nothing. I know this is not easy but with practice every day and with determination you will reach the goal. After a little time the desire to heal will come. The internal information shows how it can then happen almost by itself.

If you are already experienced in these things you can begin to use spiritual concentration to include chakra work in your meditation (see part II, 30, Vibration and elementary energy).

It makes sense to take a meditation course or seminar with experienced people. They have learnt to pass on energies with love and compassion in order to activate healing processes. This energy transfer is free (see footnotes for information). Anyone can learn to do it. With a little practice you will be able to use it on yourself or other people.

An alkaline lifestyle and the detoxification of the body described

above form a basis which strengthens the responsiveness to these
spiritual possibilities. The elementary energy of the universe is
available for free; it is simply there. Be open to new ways of thinking
and new ideas.
Today, after many years of training, I am delighted to provide help
and support to accompany the people in my seminars on the path to
healing.[48, 49]


## 17. Psychotherapy

From my own experience and from what other Parkinson's sufferers
have told me, I know that the triggers of Parkinson's disease can often
be found in the patient's psyche. At least 6 out of 10 patients confirm
this. I think that it is realistic to talk of 8 to 10 patients, as not
everyone recognises the connection or is willing to accept it.
At the very beginning of this book I talk about the similarities
between Parkinson's sufferers. I believe that psychological illnesses
are one of the parallels.

We reflect on the beginnings of our disease; we start looking for
the causes:
What makes us ill?
What makes us scared?
What makes our hands shake?
When did our knees give out for the first time?
When did we become unsteady on our feet?
Why do I always veer to the right (or left) when I walk?
When did I start putting more weight on the outside edges of my
feet (wearing down my shoes)?
When did my fears become ridiculous?
Why am I usually so sad?
Why was I suddenly unable and unwilling to drive?
When did my voice become hoarse?
When did I start feeling so old?

When did this ringing in my ears start?
Why am I not taken seriously?
Why do I break out in sweat on my head and neck, particularly at night?
Why am I so hectic, scared and resigned at the same time?
Why can't I remember people's names when I am speaking to them, even when I've known them for years?
What discussions bring on these bad headaches?
Why am I getting shorter?
When will I no longer to be able to get up and go to work?
Why do I just want my peace and quiet?
When did I develop this strong desire to be outside when the sun is shining?
Why can I no longer collect my thoughts without feeling like everything is contracting inside my head?
When did my head stop understanding what I read in the newspaper?
When was the first time that I could not find the words to give a qualified answer?
How long have I been afraid of the dark?
When did I start seeing ghosts?
Why am I suddenly no longer able to smell?
Why am I suddenly unable to swallow properly?
When did I want to end by life?
Why does water collect so unpleasantly in my mouth when I speak?
How long have I been unable to climb stairs?
Why can I no longer dress and undress on my own?
Why do I suddenly fall more often?
Why do people no longer understand me when I speak?
When did I stop caring about anything?
Etc., etc., etc. ...

The first clear signs are a slowing down of the body and brain.
You feel like you age by a year every month. The fear that you can no longer do anything is indescribable. You turn down activities of any kind. A need to be left in peace spreads within you.

Ask yourself questions that apply to you in particular as well. Date and sort these occurrences. Try to come to an honest conclusion for yourself. If you are able – and I hope with all my heart that you are – to find this special point of realisation, there is nothing better. You can accept your disease with all your love. You can experience the full effect of the therapies. Do not evaluate, simply accept. The Catholic reader will probably understand when I say that it feels the same as the relief you felt as a child after confession, like your small soul could breathe out again. This feeling that from now on everything will get better is simply indescribable and deserves to be put into practice immediately!
I therefore want to try to understand these triggers of my disease as something good. This usually does not happen right away. Be patient with yourself. Once you have recognised the problem it can only get better. In anthroposophic medicine, Professor Volker Fintelmann talks of a mental block which happens here.[50, 51] It is only later that a physical block appears as a visible expression of the disease. This explanation was crucial for me; I could suddenly answer 'when' and 'why'.
My experience was that the first of the events and questions listed above occurred around the end of 2000 and became more severe in spring 2003. However, it was not until autumn 2004 that I was diagnosed with Parkinson's disease and not until early 2006 that this was confirmed by a court.

It is important to think everything over carefully in order to determine the point when the disease began, which may be on a specific day, or after a specific event or discussion with your family or at work. If you are able to say a prayer or meditate before considering this you will soon be led to this specific point. Others find it more difficult and require professional assistance. In this case, please contact an experienced psychotherapist. Hopefully this will mean that you have the support of a wonderful person and listener, as I have found. I am very grateful to him.


## 18. Eating and living healthily

It is time to do something good and healthy for yourself and for your family! The result is worth it, as the result of your actions will be improving the entire family's health. Being healthy means being free of toxins and acids![52]

Artificially created vitamins: Every year, over 10 million people worldwide develop cancer. Around one third of cancers are proven to be linked to diet. Around 90 percent of deaths due to oesophageal, stomach and colon cancer are caused by diet.[53] These are the findings of hundreds of researchers who met at the American Heart Association's annual congress in Orlando, Florida, in November 2009. One researcher from Denmark presented an analysis of 47 clinical studies on vitamins. The result: artificially created vitamins can shorten our lives. And that is putting it nicely.

Natural diet: I have already spoken about the great importance of diet. However, I will mention it again explicitly here. Milk robs us of calcium. Milk is not as good for our children as advertising wants us to believe.[54] We should also be warned against eating cheese that contains added potassium nitrate. For all milk and cheese products, make sure that you only buy unpasteurised products. This allows us to benefit from the minerals.
The effects of minerals in milk products that have been pasteurised or thermally treated is reduced. All diet products with less than 3 percent fat should also be avoided. The body needs at least 2 percent fat in order to transport vitamins and minerals.[55] Products

containing lactobacilli can make the intestine 'addicted'. According
to current studies, normal yoghurt is just as effective.

The first thing to pay careful attention to is the raw materials used to
produce food. They must be natural and should not be genetically
modified or produced in a way that uses genetic modification
technology. They must be processed without any chemical or
synthetic additives and preservatives. They must not contain
hydrogenated fats, artificial flavour enhancers, chemical aromas or
colourings.
Nowadays most food contains ultraviolet, radioactive or ionised
radiation or ingredients that are subject to radiation during
production. These products are not real food, they simply fill us up
and make us sick or are of only limited nutritional value.
Nobody needs this rubbish, but everyone buys it and swallows it because
they do not think it is bad – or they simply do not think. What kind of
parent sends their child to school without a proper breakfast? Maybe they
have a swig of cola from the refrigerator and then off to school they go...

A good diet is part of culture. What people learn in their childhood and
during their youth under their parents roofs will shape their lives, at
the very latest when they have children themselves. Then their
memories of their own childhood come back. The memory of a mug of
hot cocoa, chicory coffee, or herbal tea can pass on the feeling of
warmth and security that we have experienced ourselves for a lifetime.
In principle, all children can be encouraged to enjoy things, even fruit
and vegetables. Top chefs and other people have been promoting this
subject with great success. Of course, parents and teachers must be
included in this campaign. This is also generally successful.
Some people are setting a good example. Good food is not
necessarily a question of cost. Often the person doing the shopping
needs to break old habits, as it requires a different kind of logistical
effort but does not cost any more.

Instead of tinned and ready-made products, please only use fresh products from the market. It is worth it. France is a great example here. They only accept the best for their children! The television channel VOX did an experiment. Children's performance was tested after they had eaten fast food and food cooked by a Michelin star chef for lunch. The result: the healthy food made from fresh products that were rich in vitamins increased their mental capacity from 42 to 61 percent. Amazingly, their ability to concentrate rose from 33 to 79 percent. The head teachers said that the children thought eating healthily was really cool.

As with anything, we must set an example to our children. Health and healthy eating should be a separate school subject. If we eat and drink tinned food, ready meals, tinned soup, crisps, cola, fizzy drinks, processed meat products and intensively farmed meat, we should not wonder if our children are overweight or if they are hyperactive and cannot concentrate at school.[56]

It is not the buzzwords like 'depression = sad because of sugar', 'addiction = caused by fat' or 'aggression = anger due to lack of vitamins' that should alarm us most.
We are responsible, the parents. Children cannot help it if they have been fed sweets and chocolate, sugary drinks with chemicals and phosphoric acid, and processed meat products until they become ill. But advertising is effective. It suggests that we can have a clear conscience; that we can sit back on the sofa, smoke a cigarette, have a beer as well and maybe a glass of schnapps and a packet of crisps to finish off a day of watching television.

These are trends that we all follow, and we do not notice the effects on our children until they are seven or eight years old. This is definitely too late. All school children in Germany could be given free fruit and vegetables at break time. The European Union in Brussels gives us money for this. The EU subsidies it with a scheme for free

fruit and vegetables for school children in Europe which has a budget of 20 million euros.[57]
When we consider that one in two children in Germany comes from a family that is on benefits, this would be a great thing. One in nine girls and one in six boys are seriously overweight. The EU has realised that something must change. In Germany, however, schools are run by the individual states and there are no politicians who wish to implement the project. The states can also apply for and receive subsidies from Brussels themselves. This works fantastically in 71 schools in the state of Saarland, for example. None of the other states are doing anything. The EU only provides money if the state matches it. With the exception of those in Saarland, state politicians are not prepared to accept this generous offer. However, the school fruit scheme has been running in 21 EU countries for a while now. Germany does not participate because state politicians prevent it from doing so. The statistics explain this. More than 30 percent of all meals that are consumed in German households are ready meals. Ready-made products are used in more than 50 percent of meals. Why is no one interested in learning what exactly it is that they are eating?

The problem of recognising and, if necessary, banning nanoparticles in food remains entirely unsolved. Our bodies are put at great risk by these particles that the industry is allowed to add to our food in uncontrolled amounts, because nanoparticles are easily absorbed by our cells. Industrial products such as chocolate bars and sweets are often covered with a nanometre-thin layer of titanium dioxide so that they no longer develop white edges, such as when they are stored incorrectly.[58] The market is booming; the food 'tastes better', lasts much longer and has a different consistency, such as ketchup which is made thicker by adding silicon dioxide.[59] Or the well-known aluminium silicate nanoparticles that stop powders caking. These mixtures have been added to packet soups and herbs for a while now in uncontrolled amounts.
Yet no one seems to be interested in the horrendous effects that

these substances can have on our cells, our blood and our organs. Ready-made pizza is coated with nanoparticles so that, depending on the heat of the microwave, it gets the taste of spinach pizza at 400 °C or tomato pizza at 800 °C, for example.[60] Nano-sized ceramic particles allow frying fat to run off chips or crisps more easily. This makes them less fatty. Sound like a good idea? But how healthy are ceramic nanoparticles?

Drink good quality still water with a pH value above 7.0 and eat fresh organic products, fruit and vegetables, with spelt bread. Ideally, if possible, bake your own whole grain spelt bread. Eat brown top millet. Brown top millet contains silicon which is important for the brain and vitamin B12 which is also essential. Long-chain omega-3 fatty acids in fish oil contain DHA and EPA which increase dopamine and serotonin levels in an unparalleled way. Cayenne pepper used as a tincture is good for the blood. The circulation is boosted much more effectively than with the pepper you can buy in the supermarket.

Be sure to avoid the E number E 330. This chemical form of citric acid is used as a preservative. It is produced chemically from the Aspergillus niger fungus. It makes the intestine wall porous; in combination with aluminium it can pass through the blood-brain barrier, settling in the brain and causing neuron damage. Or heavy metals, fungi, viruses, toxins and other substances in the intestine pass directly into the blood. For this reason, make sure you always check all E numbers carefully![61]

Sweeteners and glutamates also damage our brain cells. Make sure you do not touch them! Consuming large quantities of soya products should be avoided.[62, 63]

For a healthy future we need controlled raw materials and controlled processing according to strict quality regulations. We need proof of residues that are well below the legal limits with a clear list of all

ingredients, however small the quantities, that is easy to
understand. The chance of making this a reality remains unused. The
lobbyists are performing well. We must promote ecological projects
to encourage every family to take on this social responsibility so that
our children can live healthy lives in the future. For example, in what
is known as 'peaceable farming', the same type of crop is only
planted in a particular field once every three years. There is enough
agricultural land.

Yet further dangers that we must be aware of are lurking in our
immediate environment. Electro smog in our bedrooms which is
caused by plug sockets, televisions, mobile phones or proximity to
mobile phone masts is a potential source of disease
Geopathical factors such as water veins, faults or Hartmann grids
underneath where we sleep and work can also make us ill.

Vaccines should also be mentioned – a highly controversial topic.
These vaccines are to thank for many diseases that develop later in
life.[64, 65] There are many reasons to say no to vaccines and to see
them only as a way for the pharmaceutical industry to make money.
Flu viruses, for example, come in different types. They mutate once
every 14 days. Producing the serum and developing a vaccine against
specific viruses, on the other hand, usually takes around a year.
Children under three years of age cannot produce antibodies to
vaccine serums as their immune systems are not yet fully developed.
The common childhood diseases such as rubella and measles are
needed to strengthen the immune system. Besides this, it is a crazy
idea to inject little ones who cannot yet produce antibodies with
pathogens.
Here are a few examples:

Additives in vaccine serums[66]
Aluminium: The toxic effects of aluminium can lead to anaemia
due to decreased iron production, bone disease, osteitis due to

phosphate displacement, encephalopathy, memory problems,
language disorders, listlessness and aggression.
Aluminium hydroxide can also promote Parkinson's and Alzheimer's disease.

Mercury in the compound thiomersal has a half-life of 27 years. This
means that only half of it is broken down in this time. It is a strong
oxidising agent which increases overall cell destruction. Macrophages
at the puncture site are affected by this. In certain chemical
compounds, heavy metals like mercury can easily trigger autoimmune
reactions such as multiple sclerosis. For example, when combined with
thyroxine, a hormone produced by the thyroid gland, it can lead to
autoimmune diseases of the thyroid gland. Furthermore, mercury has
a negative effect on the production of Th1 lymphocytes. This, in turn,
increases the immune response on the hormone level. This means
that Th1 is transformed into Th2. Certain complex biochemical
processes in cell tissue increase susceptibility to allergies in
conjunction with mercury. Diseases such as Alzheimer's and
Parkinson's can also occur.

Formaldehyde: This changes the natural structure of protein which
can contribute to lymphocyte damage. Even in small concentrations
formaldehyde increases susceptibility to allergies by releasing
histamine, as has been shown in experiments.

Polymyxin B: Due to severe side effects affecting the nerves and
kidneys polymyxin B is no longer used as a therapeutic substance.
However, it is still added to vaccines.

Detailed information on flu vaccines and other vaccines is available
from the addresses given in the appendix.[67, 68, 69]

As a consequence of the damage caused by vaccines, one in one-
hundred children in the USA is now autistic. By comparison, there are
no cases of autistic children in Amish communities who reject all forms

of vaccination.[70]
Even vaccines which carry the disclaimer 'does not contain mercury' can contain mercury. The health authorities agreed with the manufacturer of a 6-in-1 vaccine for babies that the product may bear this disclaimer if no mercury is added after production. The fact that these vaccines still contain mercury is to do with the pharmaceutical company's recipe and is considered a trade secret...

Even the simplest products in our homes can harm us. We simply do not know it because advertising suggests that they are healthy or harmless. The examples below should provide an initial introduction to these everyday toxins. This list can be helpful for people with Parkinson's disease and other lifestyle diseases such as Alzheimer's disease or multiple sclerosis.
For people who are or who consider themselves healthy, they are something that is worth stopping to think about.
Heavy metals in deodorants make us ill.[71, 72, 73]
Fluoride in drinking water, toothpaste and many other products greatly damages our health.[74, 75]
Glycerine in skin creams and cosmetics damages our health.
Softening agents in soap, shampoo, toy, tools and other things damage our health.
This list could be extended indefinitely!

I pay attention to harmful substances in my daily environment, when I am shopping and especially when using the items listed above. Let us return to the example of fluoride. People with Parkinson's disease should try to consume as little fluoride, chlorine and iodine as possible. Fluoride does not protect against tooth decay![76] This fluoride is a waste product from the artificial fertilizer industry, the glass industry and the nuclear power industry. The enormous amounts that occur as the result of production in these industries were approved for the citizens of Germany back during the foundation the Republic in 1948.[77]

Fluorine does not protect against tooth decay, in fact the opposite is true: fluorine corrodes enamel and decalcifies teeth. This decalcification damages the whole body. This can lead to other diseases and susceptibility to injury, such as osteoporosis, ADD/ADHD, Alzheimer's disease, allergies, rheumatism, hip fractures and reduced intelligence. Publications by responsible dentists and researchers (see footnotes) show: fluoride is highly poisonous! It does not belong in the body. For more information see: [78, 79, 80, 81]

The home: Modern furniture, wood panelling and similar items usually contain formaldehyde. The foam in upholstered furniture is produced using chemical processes with hundreds of harmful substances, as are washing powder and cleaning materials. The insect repellents and moth repellents that we like to use are also poisonous to humans, as are weed killers. Look out for mould and yeast fungi in your home. Aspergillus niger can be found on the rubber seal in refrigerators or around the bath. Others lurk in cellars, in dishcloths, flower pots and toothbrushes, as well as in bottles that are reused. Harmful fungi can even be settled in new beer or wine bottles when you buy them.[82]

Everything that contains harmful substances must be thrown out. You cannot become healthy otherwise. I know it sounds radical, but you should decide where your priorities lie.

Laptop: Are you familiar with the photos in magazines of teenagers, children, pregnant women and other people using laptops balanced on their knees? The instructions for many laptops explicitly state that they should never be used near the stomach as this may have harmful effects. This applies especially when using Wi-Fi. However, this radiation is present even when not using the Internet, even if you are just watching a film, for example. In pregnant women it is not just the mother who may become ill. The foetus can also suffer irreparable damage.

## 19. Relationships

*Honesty in relationships:* The most important thing in any family should be honesty in the relationships. Life is full of changes. However, changes are related to one another. This forms a circle in our unconscious mind. According to Ayurvedic teaching, our lives go beyond birth and death. As Dr Vasant Lad explains, the teaching of Ayurveda place great importance on the relationships between husband and wife, father and daughter, mother and son, brother and sister, etc.[83] All relationships must contain honesty and clarity. Clarity in a relationship promotes compassion. Compassion is love. Love is clarity, and clarity is achieved through communication. Do not wear a mask in your relationships; be honest and open with one another.

Nowadays, many people lead a health-conscious lifestyle. Many are vegetarians, do yoga or exercise regularly. They look at the composition of food, with vitamins, minerals, protein, etc. However, many are still unable to heal.

This is because they focus on these small areas which, while they are important on a detailed level, are only small tiles in the great mosaic of health and healing.

Life's relationships, simply between people – starting with family and then friends, colleagues, neighbours, people we meet in public, and so on – are more important than all of these fragments, more important than any diet. Relationships are the foundation of our health, our happiness and our lifespans.

Learn to be aware of your reactions in your everyday life. Learn to perceive your consciousness in action. If your path in life is righteous it will be valuable and promote healing. Through this consciousness you will become your own light. This light will never go out.

This light is love,

this light is compassion,

this light is a pure relationship.

With regard to this I remember a presentation at a health conference
by a Dr Bösch from Switzerland. His urgent recommendation was
'reconcile yourself!'
First reconcile yourself with yourself.
Reconcile yourself with your partner.
Reconcile yourself with your children.
Reconcile yourself with your friends,
but also with your enemies.

It is not important whether these people want to be reconciled with
you or ever will be. The will for reconciliation is what matters. I have
spoken several times of a mental block, a lack of will, in Parkinson's
sufferers. When speaking to other sufferers I have found that this
mental block is often not caused by being overwhelmed at work but
is a result of a broken relationship with a partner and/or children. As
Hans Deidenbach once said, we cannot come to terms with ourselves
as long as we remain fixated on the 'wrong' that we believe others
have done to us or genuinely have done to us. To forgive, he
continued, is not to forget or supress. It is about processing
memories so we can finally be free of them.
'Genuine forgiveness does not deny anger but faces it head-on. If I
can feel outrage at the injustice I have suffered, can recognise my
persecution as such, and can acknowledge and hate my persecutor for
what he or she has done, only then will the way to forgiveness be
open to me.' (Alice Miller)


## 20. Maria Treben's therapy

Maria Treben includes two passages on Parkinson's disease in her
book *Health through God's Pharmacy*. She offers a recipe to alleviate
or even cure Parkinson's disease. She recommends wood sorrel.[84]
Maria Treben is famous for her Swedish bitters, a tonic made with
high-proof alcohol and a wide range of herbs. Swedish bitters is a

truly wonderful, diverse medicine. Maria Treben took the recipe from a Swedish doctor and popularised it in other countries. Parkinson's patients should place a compress with Swedish bitters on the back of the head for two to four hours a day, in a way that still allows them to move freely around the house. I can confirm the excellent effects and highly recommend this method of treatment.[85]
Parkinson's suffers are known to experience a general stiffness in their limbs. Maria Treben recommends thyme baths for this. These baths strengthen the muscles. However, one bath is not a magic cure; I took one bath a week for a while.[86]


## 21. Water crystals

The researcher Masaru Emoto began studying the energetic structure of water in the mid-1980s.[87] Water is not obviously directly linked to disease, but if we consider Parkinson's disease as a psychological disorder then perhaps it actually is.
On the one hand, since Einstein we have known that everything is made of energy. Masaru Emoto evaluated the energy of different types of water scientifically. In doing so, to put it simply, he came to the conclusion that it is essential for humans not only to drink good, high-quality water but for this to be energised water.
I found one of Emoto's experiments rather unsettling. He exposed a glass of water to pieces of music by Mozart and Bach, and this resulted in wonderful structures in this water.
Conversely, he exposed some water to heavy metal music or insulted it. This resulted in broken structures. If a glass of water reacts like this, I wonder what happens in our children's small bodies which, like all humans, are made of over 70 percent water? How do our loved-ones' souls react when we shout or swear at them?
Children cannot help their behaviour; often they have simply copied it from their parents. Or it is a cry for help and an attempt to get attention. Therapy has to start with the parents. Children need to be given clear guidelines on how to behave. If parents are too weak or

busy to give their children clear rules, they should not be surprised when their children react by screaming.

Water that can be collected from the surface has considerably more energy than water that has been pumped up many metres and squeezed through pipes. This means that our tap water is of rather low quality in comparison with energised water, although it varies from region to region. I have determined very poor energy values in some regions, which was probably due to PFT pollution.
As I have mentioned earlier, the easiest way to energise tap water is with a spring water generator, which is installed directly after the water meter in the water supply to your home. The water is then immediately suitable for household use at least. However, I only use pure spring water for drinking and preparing food.


## 22. Healing water

The most effective, natural and direct form of energised water can be found in healing springs, such as those at pilgrimage sites. This water is of course still healing water without the spiritual background simply due to its physical and biochemical composition. However, I like to acknowledge the spiritual background and always use healing water in conjunction with a short prayer or peaceful and loving thoughts.
Ever since my pilgrimage to Lourdes, I have been drinking one glass of this healing water every day for the benefit of my organs and I massage my head with this wonderful water to help my brain in particular to become healthy again. The water from Lourdes is especially good for strengthening the entire immune system. It can be ordered from Lourdes.

From my research I know that water from Fatima has proven to be particularly helpful for diseases of the brain. The resonance and energy of this healing water mainly influence the cerebrum.
Montichiari water from the famous pilgrimage site in Italy near Brescia

is good for the metabolism and cell growth. Medjugorje water from Bosnia and Herzegovina has a unique effect on the immune system. San Damiano water from Piedmont near Piacenza is used for the immune system and also benefits the cerebrum.[88, 89]
The most famous source of healing water in Germany is the St Leonhardsquelle in St Stephan's church in Rosenheim. Seven variations of it are sold in health food shops. It is worth testing them and then deciding which one you think is best for your body. For Parkinson's patients, the *Lichtquelle, Sonnenquelle* and *Quelle St.Georg* variations are particularly recommended.[90]


## 23. Hildegard therapy

Saint Hildegard of Bingen lived around 850 years ago. She did not know about Parkinson's disease of course, but she knew the symptoms. Hildegard's teachings on holistic medicine are put into practice today by Dr Wighard Strehlow in Allensbach by Lake Constance in Germany.

In his book *Hildegard-Heilkunde von A bis Z* (Hildegard medicine from A to Z), Parkinson's disease is classified as a rheumatic disease, while in healing stone therapy it is listed under diseases of the brain and nerves.[91]
There are various dietary recommendations for people with Parkinson's disease, such as using celery seed powder every morning for several months.
The recipe is as follows: Mix 60g celery seed powder, 20g rue powder, 15g nutmeg powder, 10g clove powder and 5g meadow saxifrage powder and eat for breakfast on spelt bread with quince jam, chewing thoroughly.
You can go without it occasionally, but should stick to it for the majority of the time.

A mixed savoury powder is recommended for the tremor.[92] The recipe is as follows: 50g savoury, 40g sage powder and 30g cumin. Put one teaspoon of this mixture in a cup of fennel tea with 1 tablespoon of honey and 1 teaspoon or 30 drops of liquorice juice. Take once a day after a meal for 6 to 8 months.

The sensational 'nerve cookies' must not be forgotten. I recommend you find the recipe in a specialist book on Hildegard's work. However, the most important recommendation is to cut wheat products out of your diet and replace them with spelt products from now on. Hildegard's healing stone therapy recommends blue chalcedony for Parkinson's disease, a stone with fantastic properties. It soothes impatience for those who suffer from it,[93] and is also popularly known as the stone of speakers and singers. Chalcedony promotes concentration, and keeps the flow of thoughts running smoothly and the airways and bronchi free of toxins. It has also been shown to keep overacidification in check. I had a chalcedony bracelet made and can confirm the above-mentioned effects. I have been wearing it constantly ever since.
I have also had good experiences with the emerald that Hildegard recommends as a healing stone. On days when I felt that I was relapsing the emerald gave me strength. During the acute stage of my disease I always carried an emerald in the breast pocket of my shirt. When I experienced severe pain or tension in my head I simply used surgical tape to fix it to where the pain was worst.[94]
It is now possible to determine the energy of these stones scientifically using biophysics. It is measured in nanometres. This energy can also be visualised by biophoton photography, which makes the electromagnetic radiation visible.

Please do not be put off by people who, for whatever reason, question the healing energy of precious stones. Make up your own mind.


## 24. Rechtsregulat

Rechtsregulat is a liquid created through fermentation that provides the body with accessible enzymes. It completes the body's own stock of enzymes. This leads to more antibodies being produced and takes strain off the body.

One possible dosage is to take one tablespoon of Rechtsregulat (do not use a metal spoon) in the morning before eating and in the evening before going to sleep and hold it in your mouth for a long time (up to five minutes). By doing this the enzymes in it are absorbed by the oral mucosa.

The advantage of Rechtsregulat compared to other enzymes is the variety of ingredients used to make it. Since the 1990s, more and more studies have shown that secondary plant substances, including phytovitamins, are very important for the body's enzyme production. They cannot be produced artificially. Macromolecules such as enzymes and proteins are made accessible. Only natural organic ingredients such as lemons, dates, walnuts, figs, coconuts, soya beans, sprouts, celery, artichokes, millet, peas and saffron are used for the fermentation process.

The company Dr. Niedermaier Pharma has developed a special process called cascade fermentation that meets high quality standards and does not use preservatives, chemical additives, added sugar, alcohol, etc.[95]

What is cascade fermentation? It is a multi-step fermentation process in which ingredients are made accessible and soaked in dextrorotary lactic acid. This concentrates valuable components in fresh fruit, nuts and vegetables in a natural way. The resulting product supports the body, enabling it to develop its powers of regulation, immunomodulation and antioxidation.

All Rechtsregulat products are gluten-free and suitable for people with milk allergies. They have a unique biological effect that acts as a preliminary stage before the body's own enzyme production. This allows deficiencies to be rectified. The intestine is strengthened, the metabolism is improved and the immune system is supported. Rechtsregulat

products are also suitable for children, pregnant women, diabetics and people suffering from alcohol addiction. They can also be used for prophylaxis. They are a great addition to an alkaline lifestyle.
The following methods in which I use them, other than taking a tablespoon in the morning and evening, are controversial: I prepare a mixture of one part Rechtsregulat and two parts Lourdes water in a nasal spray bottle. I spray this mixture into my nose like a normal nose spray, quickly and high up in the sinuses. I have always had positive experiences using it in this way, such as before car journeys, before writing this, and whenever I need or want to concentrate particularly hard.[96]

## 25. Homeopathic therapy

In homeopathy, developed by Samuel Hahnemann (1755–1843), a thorough investigation is made to find the causes of a diseases. Hahnemann was not just a doctor; he was also a chemist and pharmacist. His approach, in which the aim is to heal not only individual areas of the body but the person as a whole, is the key principle of homeopathy.

If you pay attention to your body's signals, you will suddenly realise that certain reactions reoccur when you do certain things. For this reason, homeopathy is also known as *Erfahrungsmedizin* – literally 'experience medicine' – in German, in reference to the experiences that individuals and society as a whole have had and passed on over the centuries.

Homeopathy has many supporters around the globe. Great poets, famous thinkers, composers, popes and presidents have been healed with homeopathy. Johann Wolfgang von Goethe once wrote a passionate letter about what he described as 'the teachings of the wonderful doctor named Hahnemann.'[97].

Charles Darwin changed our idea of world history with his theory of evolution and was a client of homeopathy, as was his family. Mother Teresa worked with homeopathic globules in the streets of Calcutta. Other famous users of homeopathy include Abraham Lincoln,

Marlene Dietrich, Pope Paul VI, Charles Dickens, Vincent van Gogh,
Frederik Chopin, Karl Carstens and Richard Wagner.
The great Indian leader Mahatma Gandhi once said, 'Dr Hahnemann
was a man of superior intellectual power and means of saving human
life, having a unique medical nerve. I bow before his skill and the
Herculean and humanitarian labour he did.' Dr Hahnemann's main
rule was *similia similibus curentur* – like cures like. This approach lead
to the term 'homeopathy' (Greek: homoios = similar; pathos =
suffering). This is in contrast to conventional medicine, which can be
described as alleopathy – i.e. healing suffering through the other. Dr
Hahnemann published his first work on ascertaining the healing powers
of drugs in 1796. His most famous work, *The Organon of the Healing
Art*, was published in 1810.
At the beginning of the twentieth century, the Mayo brothers, founders
of the world-famous Mayo Clinic in the USA, hoped that one day the
public would recognise the wonderful results of homeopathy.

Although homeopathy is now well established in certain hospitals, such as
the Charité in Berlin and Essen University Hospital, it is still
regrettably met with a lack of understanding, head shaking and even
scorn by most people in conventional medicine. The first pupil of Dr
Hahnemann was a homeopath named Ordenstern who began treating
Parkinson's disease with Belladonna globules in 1867.

I have seen that phosphorus and caustrum, for example, also list
many symptoms of Parkinson's disease under their therapeutic
indications. Parkinson's patients find walking and orientating
themselves particularly difficult, particularly when streets or ramps
are steep. In these cases the fear of falling is particularly great. Borox
globules can help here. Carbo animalis can also provide psychological
support to help overcome long-term problems, possibly in
combination with Hura brasilensis.
However, I have deliberately not provided information about the
strength and dosage of the globules, as these should be determined

by an experienced homeopath. Please also pay attention to them yourself for the benefit of your healing.

Why is homeopathy not widely accepted? In my opinion, one of the reasons is that it is not expensive – it is not possible to make a lot of money out of it. Try comparing the Bovis value of homeopathic medicines with your medications. A simple small arnica globule with a strength of C30 has a Bovis value of around 64 000 BU. In addition, when homeopathy is used properly there are no toxic side effects like there are from the pharmaceutical industry's offerings. The aim of homeopathy is to keep its patients healthy for many years and allow them to be healthy as they grow old healthily.


## 26. Anthroposophic therapy

Anthroposophy and anthroposophic medicine were strictly forbidden by the governments in Germany and Austria during the Second World War. Only a small group of around 100 anthroposophic practitioners were allowed to live and work in exile in the German-speaking part of Switzerland.
Anthroposophic medicine combines a scientific and a philosophical approach that, in addition to the physical parts of the body, also considers the spiritual structures. Anthroposophy speaks of four dimensions of the body. Dr Rudolf Steiner (1861–1925), the founder of anthroposophy, called them the physical body, the etheric body, the astral body and the ego. Anthroposophy made the first steps towards treating people in the 1920s at the initiative of the Dutch doctor Ita Wegmann (1876–1943) who was famous for showing how anthroposophy could enrich medicine.

Anthroposophic medicine describes the real cause of Parkinson's disease as a mental block. Disruptions to movements are the consequence of this. The mind is willing but the consciousness is not able to put what it wants into practice effectively. Recognising this connection is crucial in order to develop a treatment plan.

Parkinson's patients need to carry out exercises of will, accompanied by power of expression and feelings such as happiness, interest and compassion. Prayer and/or meditation can also be used as exercises of will in this context.
Movement, movement, movement is the most important thing for the body here. Each time a patient goes for a walk, consciously being aware of nature, it promotes their powers of self-healing.

Diet should be chosen carefully and should be balanced. Fruit, leaves and seeds are ideal. The amount of root vegetables, meat and fish should be limited and milk should only be in the form of fermented milk. Take care with coffee, tea and alcohol. All kinds of drugs, including tobacco, should be avoided, as should spirits.

Artistic activities also train the will. This is incredibly important for Parkinson's patients. Combining movement with music is ideal. Dancing is also a form of physiotherapy. Carrying out artistic activities helps us fight our disease.

Rhythmic massages and massages using oils as developed by Wegmann/Hauschka are used for Parkinson's disease. Some recommendations include St John's wort oil in the morning and lavender oil at night, as well as strong iron ointment and highly concentrated zinc ointment that are rubbed into the skin rhythmically in the area around the liver. There are also a wide range of anthroposophic medicines that can be used on an individual basis to treat Parkinson' sufferers. The aim of these medicines is to stimulate the harmonic interaction of the physical and spiritual body at its centre – the liver.

The iron and zinc ointments mentioned above aim to promote bile flow, thereby supporting the aspect of will of the liver function. Iron is administered orally with celandine. In addition to the zinc ointment, which is used externally, zinc injections support the body's constructive processes. Zinc helps ensure smooth movements; this effect is improved with the addition of honey. If a patient's mental (cognitive) abilities are particularly affected, a preparation of strong lead with honey is used. The ego and the will are stimulated by strong plant and animal venoms.

Althropa/deadly nightshade extracts and datura toxins are mentioned here (datura is also used in healing mixtures in Indian healing plant therapies). These substances must be prescribed by a doctor and must only be used under medical supervision. For this reason, I will not provide details of dosages or strengths here.
Preparation of the recipes and treatment should of course be done by an anthroposophic doctor.

Discussion with the patient is particularly important in anthroposophic medicine. Based on the teachings of Asclepius, the famous doctor of Greek Antiquity, Hippocrates, a scholar of his, posited that the word must always be the first step towards therapy. Personal history, an investigation of the root causes of disease, and consideration of further developments and goals are therefore the centre of attention for Parkinson's patients. Religious aspects of the patient's life and their experiences are also considered in these discussions, even if this topic might seem very personal to some people.
What binds the patient and the anthroposophic doctor is the practical experience of the words of Christ: 'For where two or three are gathered together in my name, there am I in the midst of them.' A person who chooses to live their life in freedom and with joy will be able to recognise their own strengths better, learn to love them and understand them as a motivation. The Parkinson's patient must therefore do much more than simply take the prescribed medicine when undergoing anthroposophic therapy. They must be active themselves in order to overcome their disease and to recognise that

disease is not an unalterable fate.

Anthroposophic medicine asks what came before birth and what will come after death. These questions concerning the meaning of life and disease are becoming more and more important in the therapies, especially with the goal of finding qualified answers.[98, 99, 100]

For me these thoughts were a fundamental realisation. If the liver is not healthy it is not possible to cure Parkinson's disease, because according to anthroposophy the liver is the organ of will. The liver is the location of our life force in the true sense of the world. The word 'liver' contains the word 'live'. I therefore recommend having your blood examined using dark field microscopy, followed by diagnosis and detoxification using homeopathic methods.
I do not know a single Parkinson's sufferer whose liver does not display considerable damage and toxification due to heavy metals, viruses, fungi, acids, worms, bacteria and, above all, medication. Medicines for rheumatic diseases, antidepressants and pain medication in general are particularly bad for the liver, gall bladder and kidneys. Consuming industrial sugar, glucose, white flour, coffee, fizzy drinks, fried food, chemical additives, tobacco, alcohol and the like also has its effects.
The first reaction to this toxification is headaches. Later comes severe tiredness that sometimes comes suddenly and is sometimes a permanent expression of excessive strain on the liver. Next comes listlessness. You no longer want to go out and withdraw from family life and society. These are symptoms of Parkinson's disease.

I strongly recommend the following: Carry out gall bladder and liver purification (see, for example, Dr Clark's[101] and Martin Frischknecht's[102] methods) and kidney purification (using Breuss' method[103]) once or twice a year to remove the toxins that have accumulated. With an alkaline lifestyle it is then possible to keep the organs more or less free of these harmful substances. To be on the safe side, I also take ground clinoptilolite once or twice a week before going to bed to remove the toxins that have accumulated or come free.

There are also other aspects to consider. Parkinson's disease and many other diseases are not purely due to modern nutrition. Other causes include eating habits, such as eating too quickly when stressed and angry or eating mindlessly in front of the television. Incidentally, patients who have had gall bladder operations are often more likely to suffer from the symptoms mentioned above. The body needs bile in the liver and intestine. If there is a lack of bile, the liver has a much harder job trying to maintain the health of the body.
The problem is that blood tests carried out as part of routine check-ups often display normal liver values. There are no tests in conventional medicine that can confirm whether the bile ducts in the liver are free or blocked by toxins and deposits. Liver diseases can only be confirmed with gamma-GT after severe damage has become apparent. Unfortunately, conventional medicine is usually not interested in possible natural detoxification methods. This is a shame, as it would mean many operations could be avoided.


## 27. Lymph therapy

When I first heard that I could activate the lymph fluid in my head using a special treatment, to be honest I was not sure what that meant. However, after I had had a session of treatment with a specially training physiotherapist I began to understand.

To start with the treatment felt a little strange. I found it uncomfortable to have a stranger wearing silicone gloves working in my mouth. By the second or third session I tried to be aware of which areas of my mouth were being worked on. The differences lie in the intensity and the type of movements, which can be in circles, in spirals, smoothing motions or movements with gentle, pump-like pressure. I am now able to practice these techniques everyday by myself.

It was some time before I began to use other measures to support this therapy. The lymph fluid is kept in motion by bouncing on a trampoline. I should have begun using the trampoline earlier, but at the time I was unaware of the benefits. One of the functions of the lymph fluid is to ensure balance in the inner ear. If it is overburdened this may lead to dizziness and an unsteady gait. These unpleasant feelings can be remedied easily and cheaply with trampoline exercises.

But I'm getting ahead of myself. Our knowledge of the lymph system is ancient and also very simple. Doctors of conventional medicine never identified or treated the lymph as a possible cause of disease for me.

What is the function of the lymph, in general and in Parkinson's disease? Put simply, the lymph transports toxins, viruses and bacteria out of our bodies or feeds them into the blood so they can be removed later.

The body produces two to three litres of lymph fluid per day to perform these tasks. Lymph fluid is almost clear or slightly white. Around 85 percent of our bodily fluids are lymph fluid.

It is therefore clear how important it is to keep this system in motion through physical activity, but also by drinking the right amount. I suggest you drink one litre more per day than you have been drinking until now (good quality still water, alkaline tea or watered-down fruit or vegetable juice). Your circulation and nerve tissue will benefit directly from this.

Once deposits have formed due to germs and toxins, the lymph does not work properly. The toxins are no longer removed but are deposited in the tissue, in the organs, and in the nerve tissue of the brain. This leads to well-known diseases. Sufficient movement also influences the essential supply of oxygen to the blood. Here the relationships between the blood, oxygen, movement, connective tissue and the conductivity of the nervous system are clear.[104]

The lymph system has around 600 lymph nodes. White blood cells
are found in the lymph nodes. White blood cells ensure that invading
toxins and impurities are combated effectively. Detoxification and
purification takes place in the circulatory system and the lymph
system. This process is particularly thorough when the body is
supplied with enough oxygen and liquid.
We supply our bodies with the required oxygen by breathing. You
should be able to feel your diaphragm move as you breath good air
consciously when walking with large, strong steps, when doing sport,
when moving your head and torso, and when doing similar exercises.
Laughing is also beneficial. A hearty laugh that makes the diaphragm
shake is good for your health. If you like to laugh (without necessarily
having a reason), you can try a course of laughter yoga.

Another option is to add $H_2O_2$ (3% hydrogen peroxide = liquid
oxygen) to high quality drinking water.[105] This provides the red blood
cells with additional oxygen. The lymph fluid must flow; patients with
brain diseases, cancer, diabetes, multiple sclerosis or polio, for
example, should have the lymph flow activated by a specialist
therapist to detoxify the cells more effectively. Good quality water
and oxygen must be supplied in all forms. Craniosacral therapy and
special forms of acupuncture promote the lymph flow.
This is all very easy. It does not cost much and is very effective.


## 28. Aslan therapy

This therapy was developed by Professor Ana Aslan (1897–1988).
The therapy was presented at the fist medical congress of its kind in
1956 and was met with much scepticism.
During many years of clinical practice, Ana Aslan collected knowledge
of the active agent procaine. Usually procaine is used for local
anaesthetic. However, Professor Aslan spent decades developing
treatment concepts for regeneration therapy to counteract wear and

ageing processes in humans.

As we age the cells in our tissues and organs lose their strength and vitality. These processes have a significant effect on what are known as free radicals. These natural waste products damage the tissue and organs, which leads to signs of wear as we age. Procaine neutralises free radicals directly in the cells where they are formed – without any harmful side effects. However, so far over 5000 research projects on Aslan therapy have been unable to explain how this happens. Professor Aslan treated people all over the world. Many famous people also regularly visit Aslan clinics.

As chance would have it, there is an Aslan clinic just a few kilometres from where I live, so I was able to find out about the treatment in detail. I began a course of outpatient therapy and was pleasantly surprised at the clinic's approach – from the initial detailed two-hour consultation with the doctor to the therapy session with the very friendly and skilled staff. I was convinced. The deciding factor for me was the holistic treatment concept that was an ideal combination of conventional and alternative medicine.

The Romanian doctor and cell biologist Ana Aslan discovered back in the 1950s that patients were livelier and more powerful after being give procaine. Results produced by research groups at the Charité in Berlin, the Spanish National Cancer Research Centre and other leading institutes have since confirmed that procaine can do much more for our health than previous thought. The first studies on the relationship between Parkinson's disease and age-related diseases were carried out in the 1960s. In addition to the known rejuvenating effects on cells, procaine was observed to cause blood vessels to dilate and to have antidepressant and antioxidant effects.

The treatment is as follows. The doctor determines the dosage for the daily procaine injection based on the patient's current needs and the additional vitamins and minerals that they require. Procaine infusions can also be used. The therapy can be complemented by a wide range of other treatments, such as physiotherapy, health therapy, medical spa treatments, light therapy or acupuncture. I also found the informative presentations, yoga courses and various other different sessions offered very pleasant.

What were the effects? As I had already tried many different therapies by then I was naturally sceptical at first. But I felt good. I coped well with everything. And I did not leave anything out. I tried everything the Aslan clinic had to offer, from professional courses on how to use Nordic walking as movement therapy to the craniosacral therapy that I appreciated greatly. My three weeks of treatment flew by. The course of therapy finished with a thorough final examination during which medications for the coming weeks were suggested, once again confirming my good impression.

Two to three weeks later I felt a positive boost going through my body and my head. I was able to concentrate better and was considerably more active. I was suddenly making plans to travel or play golf again. I simply felt able to do more. This result was beyond my expectations.

Aslan therapy is a good, solid addition to the therapies that I used and works fantastically in combination with the alkaline lifestyle, deacidification, physiotherapy, heavy metal detoxification and methods of cleansing the blood and intestine identified as a result of dark field microscopy. Thanks to its holistic concept it is absolutely to be recommended and should be integrated into treatment for Parkinson's disease.[106]

## 29. Horst Krohne's therapy

I became aware of Horst Krohne though various episodes of the television series Fliege in 2003 and 2004 shortly after I had begun to suffer from Parkinson's disease. In each episode I was very impressed

by his performance and successful healing. However, back then I did not consider this especially helpful for me. It was only later that I was shown Horst Krohne's *Handbuch für heilende Hände*[107] (handbook for healing hands) by a healer. This time I recognised that I was being presented with an opportunity, particularly after I had read a section of the book on treating Parkinson's disease. This was another place where the core problems were clearly identified. Horst Krohne begins by saying that it is highly likely that the brain's energy is being disrupted by heavy metals such as mercury. This affects all regeneration and supply meridians. There are also problems with the cervical spine. Disruption in the energy in the transformer (a subchakra), a biomagnetic field around the atlas, the top vertebra (C1), can be observed. This transformer regulates the nervous tension between the brain and the spinal cord. According to Horst Krohne, before healing therapy can begin it is essential that the body is first detoxified of heavy metals. If this is not done first the disease may become worse. The same applies to the consumption of alcohol and nicotine. Only once these substances have been removed can the reconstruction of the disrupted energy fields begin.
In his book Horst Krohne also recommends using meridian treatment and working with a spiritual guide. In this example I saw once again that I needed to get to know the possibilities of medication first before looking at other methods of healing. Later, after having learnt meditation and energy transfer techniques, I was able with a bit of practice to concentrate specifically on the topic of my spine and the edge of my skull. In some books this area is also called the subchakra or Medulla oblongata. Those who are not so experienced can place their hand on this area.

Do not be afraid, anyone can heal. We all have the power of the universe in us. With a short prayer or loving thought we can concentrate and supply this area with energy. If, despite concentrating hard, you do not believe you can do it, you should look for a healer who can go through these methods with you several times until you are able to do it yourself.

## 30. Vibration and elementary energy

$e = mc^2$. Albert Einstein proved with his formula that all matter is energy. Energy (e) = mass (m) x the speed of light (c) squared. This points to light as the link between matter and energy. Leading physicists have since proven that the universe's elementary particles, quanta, out of which everything is made, constantly send out electromagnetic waves. I know that this is a very simplified explanation but I hope it makes it clearer.

For this reason, the natural fluctuations in the Earth's magnetic field also play a role in determining our consciousness. Researchers believe that various diseases can be traced to these irregularities in the magnetic field due to the sun.

And our bodies are also vibration. They are made up of the vibration or electromagnetic waves of our billions of cells, energy that flows through our bodies, our organs, even the smallest nerve cells every millisecond. The German physicist Max Planck said that there is no matter as such; everything is made up of vibrations.

As we as humans are made of 70 to 80 percent water, the vibrations of our organs and our blood can allow us to live a healthy life, as the vibrations of humans mirrors the vibrations of the Earth.

Unfortunately, this simple view is no longer easy to put into practice. Our modern world sometimes creates levels of vibration that are millions of times higher than normal, which can disrupt our cells to a lesser or greater degree or even destroy them, leading to disease.

For example, the frequency of the Earth's magnetic field is 7.8Hz on average. This corresponds to the vibration frequency of our heart meridian. The frequency of a domestic electricity supply is around 50Hz and radio frequency is around 100MHz. Mobile phone radiation is no less than 1800MHz, while computer radiation is 2800MHz. This should make it clear how harmful and life-threatening our world has become.

The teachings of bioresonance show us how to understand these effects and integrate them into our lives so that we can be healthy in resonance with nature. Our brain wave activities are around 40Hz and are the basis of clear thoughts. The nerve cells vibrate in gamma waves. When the brain switches to creative thinking, it vibrates in alpha wave mode. Alpha waves are the natural status of consciousness for children up to seven years old. Children at this age are physically relaxed but highly active mentally and particularly observant. This is the learning phase of the first few years of life.
In the phase between going to sleep and waking up the brain of an adult is in alpha frequency. Here we experience the problems of our daily lives that we have created ourselves in our dreams. We have lived too little, loved too little; we have experienced hatred, envy, jealously and stress in all their forms. Everything returns; the brain forgets nothing. It has no sense of time. But we can learn from this: what we can do better, what we can achieve for our health with love and new ways of thinking. A wonderful experience. Biophysicists can see these connections clearly.

Disease is always related to disregard for natural approaches to life such as love, compassion, honesty and many more factors – whether this happens consciously, unintentionally or as a matter of habit.
The frequencies of brain waves represent different mental states. Slow delta waves, for example, are characteristic of deep sleep, when the self-healing powers of our bodies are fully activated. Alpha waves with around 10Hz also occur in a relaxed state when we are awake; gamma waves with over 30Hz occur during high cognitive performance or in moments of absolute concentration.
Attentiveness and concentration, but also fear, stress and excitement, correspond to beta waves and should, if necessary, be treated by a specialist therapist. For example, through meditation that guides and influences the theta waves in the brain, these states can be improved, particularly in the case of disease.

Brain waves in the theta rhythm cause dream-like states and, when used in a therapeutic way, are an effective method of improving the quality of life for patients with disease, accelerating the healing of wounds and bones, etc.

Disease is a lack of energy (energy = vibration).

Disease is a result of incorrect, low vibrations and, in some cases, frequencies that are too high. Professor A. W. Harvey recommends slow music by Bach, Vivaldi or Handel for Parkinson's patients.[108] This music has a particularly relaxing effect or stimulates active relaxation in the creative phase, as its tempo is slower than our heart beat. The brain then switches to absorption mode. As all of this is neither difficult nor expensive, conventional medicine likes to laugh at these methods of treatment or even declare that they are harmful.
However, there are now many doctors who have used these methods of healing successfully themselves with members of their own families (although usually only them). Hopefully this will spread gradually.

As Albert Einstein said, problems cannot be solved by the same level of thinking that created them.
So let us finally recognise that we can only help ourselves. Let us finally recognise the divinity within us. Let us accept it so that we can help ourselves to become healthy again. Only we can help ourselves! The secret of healing is bound together with the principle of guided meditation. The crucial thing here is the inner pictures, the belief in a bigger picture.
At the level of the brain each of us still has the knowledge from the beginnings of humankind. It is the knowledge of the healing methods that have been used for thousands of years or were used thousands of years ago. It is healing through meditation and through the laying of hands.

It is very important to me to introduce people to the possibilities of

elementary medicine.[109]
I wish everyone, especially those affected by disease, the openness and preparedness to accept this wonderful form of energy to support the healing process effectively for the long-term. The method is simply unique. As I have already mentioned, over the course of my disease I investigated and considered different types of energy transfer and their content in seminars. In addition to the meditation style developed by Dr Shioya that I discovered in 2009, there are many other techniques. On the basis of these very different experiences I decided to use only elementary meditation for myself. It very quickly improves concentration, gets rid of stress, strengthens the immune system and promotes your mental development and that of those around you. It influences problems in the body. It is of course always better to stabilise health as a preventative measure and to use meditation to relieve or prevent stress. As the body, mind and soul are one unit, when using these techniques you should look out for improvements in your physical health too.
The diverse possibilities of elementary meditation can easily be integrated into your daily life; the technique is easy for anyone to learn. After a weekend seminar you will already be able to help yourself and your family.
In more advanced seminars on elementary medicine you can learn techniques that increase perception and concentration through meditation and energy transfer in order to improve the quality of life and work for yourself and those around you. In this context, I remain true to a Tibetan proverb: do not seek to follow in the footsteps of the masters; seek what they sought!

In conventional medicine, fungi, viruses and similar are killed with antibiotics and other chemical preparations with low vibrations. In homeopathic medicine, these things are removed from the body using natural products with highly energetic vibrations. Through energy transfer, however, strong vibrations reach the whole body immediately and stimulate the healing process directly at the cellular level. I am incredibly thankful for this possibility of healing and I am convinced that years of meditation have made a crucial contribution to my new, healthy life – through both the direct influence on my organs and the supportive psychological guidance.

I am especially glad to be able to pass on this knowledge and these personal experiences in my regular seminars.[110] In principle, everyone can activate their powers of self-healing.

Over the past few years, I have learnt to recognise different kinds of vibrations and use them for myself. It began during the worst time in 2005 and 2006 when my body had its lowest vibration of only around 1900 to 2000 Bovis units.
The knowledge of the vibrations of singing bowls, the subtle vibrations of homeopathic medicine, Schüßler salts, healing stones and the vibrations of my food, my home and everything else now determines my daily life. All that is required then is a small step in meditation with God or with a higher being of your own faith or with the universe to feel the strongest and purest vibrations.
Therefore, we should start by considering the things that are very easy to change when we are sick: our homes, where we sleep and our food. We must be able to feel completely comfortable in our homes. Many Parkinson's patients find that the place where they sleep is disrupted by earth radiation and/or electro smog. This must be corrected.
The easiest way to determine that there is a disruption is if you feel more at ease when you go on a trip than when you are at home. This means that something is not right. A simple way of finding out whether the place where you sleep is disrupted in some way is with a simple compass. Place it on the mattress then slide it very slowly over the whole bed. If the needle moves around restlessly in certain areas this means there is a disruption. You can then get a professional geophysicist to look for the cause.

We should also surround ourselves with things with high vibrations, such as healing stones, healing crystals, herbs and healing water. In Tibet, vibrations have been used for healing for thousands of years. When people develop a specific disease they look for a specific monastery with a special bell that hangs in a room. For a different disease there is a different monastery with a corresponding bell. The people with the disease gather around the bell. The bell is rung. The tolling of the bell, its vibration, that is sent out unto the room gives the body information. The body's own vibrations absorb the bell's vibrations to activate its powers of self-healing. The people with the disease sometime stay in these rooms for several days.
The same thing happens on a small scale with singing bowl therapy. We also speak of a feeling of vibration in our personal relationships when we recognise that another person is 'on the same wave length'. We should simply surround ourselves with people who are on the same wave length as us.

The next step applies to our food and drink. Make sure you only consume food and drink that has high vibrations.
These include organic fruit and vegetables, spelt products, pure honey, pure water and fruit juice, herbs and herbal teas; all things with good and high Bovis values. If you do not know how to use a pendulum yourself please ask someone who does. I am sure they will be happy to help. If the values measured by the pendulum do not seem believable they can be confirmed by a biophysics laboratory. Values are then given in nanometres (nm). One nanometre is equivalent to around 10 Bovis units (BU).
Around 2500 years ago, Hippocrates said: let food be your medicine and medicine be your food.
It has been this easy for thousands of years. Why don't we think of it? Because it is too easy? These wonderful findings will manifest themselves in your body after a little time. Your body's vibration will increase because you will heal, slowly but surely. You can grow old healthily in this way. With regard to the average age of the

population, people who live with God such as priests, pastors and people who live in monasteries are well ahead in the statistics. I believe that this is due firstly to the fact that these people (at least the ones I know) easy a very balanced diet. Food grown in monasteries has high levels of vibration. This is complemented by selected hand-processed foods, etc. The set fasting days are naturally also good for their health. These people eat very consciously. Secondly, whether priests or monks, these people usually live in church buildings such as monasteries or rectories that are attached or close to churches. Churches always have a high level of vibration that usually only changes or normalises at a distance of several metres. Our churches – or at least the old ones that were built by architects with geomantic knowledge – are built on sites with high vibrations, often the holy sites of our ancestors. There were very high vibrations in these places even before the buildings were constructed. Excellent examples of this include the cathedrals in Chartres and Cologne, and many more.

Today most of us do not live in holy buildings and we cannot get our food from the gardens of monasteries. We usually eat what the supermarkets are currently offering. For this reason, it is particularly important to refrain from eating the things that already have low, sometime harmful vibrations.

Over time we learn to make distinctions and only eat and drink products with high vibrations that support the body's self-healing processes directly and allow us to become healthy again. However, we should also learn that we cannot determine everything ourselves. We are exposed to the circumstances of the universe, such as the sun with its influences on the Earth's magnetic field. Yet we can be conscious of what healing means; what it means to develop these vibrations in ourselves until we can say that we are    healthy again.

To experience this healing, even when it can only be felt in small steps to start with, is something to be deeply thankful for. We can say thank you to the people who have helped us to recognise what we need to recognise. We can thank the people who have helped us with our therapies and methods. And we can say thank you to he who has healed us. Only HE can; nothing can be done without his help.

For me it is truly the most wonderful thing to say a prayer of thanks to God – or whatever you want to call him – from the bottom of my heart. Anyone can and should do this according to their own faith or in a way that is suitable for them. It is really very easy, as there is only ONE, regardless of what you call him. In this thanks we and our souls experience the highest level of vibration that we can reach. This is full of unending love; full of peace for the Earth and for all people. This has an effect on the body, the mind and the soul.


## 31. Order therapies

As I have already described, I had the opportunity to test various zappers. It began in 2006 with the Dr Clark Full Gamma Generator from the USA that was new at the time. This zapper was developed by Dr Hulda Clark to recognise and remove things in the body that cause disease, such as parasites, viruses and bacteria, especially the different worms in the intestine, liver and pancreas.[111] Hulda Clark has also been successful at treating cancer, HIV/AIDS, tumours, diabetes and other diseases and has developed so-called programme drivers for various specific diseases to treat everything from acne and Alzheimer's disease to teeth and cysts. Furthermore, the accompanying documentation is clear and includes helpful descriptions and illustrations.

Dr Clark's liver cleanse, which naturally removes gall stones without surgery, is unbeatable. Other therapists have also used her method. In this context I also learnt about the Munich-based alternative practitioner A. E. Baklayan who deepens the knowledge of these things in his book *Parasiten – die verborgene Ursache vieler*

*Erkrankungen* (parasites – the hidden cause of many diseases). I was given the chip or programme driver for Parkinson's disease by a friend. I initially used it very carefully and slowly increased the duration of treatment to the recommended time. Unfortunately, it was difficult for me to use it in the long-term as I experienced many problems and a feeling of pressure on the back left of my head. For this reason, I only used the device on the lowest setting and later only used it every few months for three weeks at a time. In 2009, I found out about the Power Quick Zap and PowerTube from a friend in Switzerland. These are devices that work in a similar way to TENS devices (TENS = transcutaneous electrical nerve stimulation) for lay people. They were constructed by the Swiss electrical engineer Martin Frischknecht, essentially based on the findings of Dr Clark but more technically developed.[112]

After I had the opportunity to test the Power Quick Zap over a longer period of time I was very satisfied. It was only later that I read in various specialist books and reports from alternative practitioners about the success of these types of devices developed by Martin Frischknecht. Uwe Karstädt reports in his book *Entgiften statt vergiften* (detoxification instead of toxification) that, by homogenising the molecular cell structures, the Power Quick Zap helps to restore unity and order. The device emits vibrations on three basic frequencies with a corresponding overtone scale which creates an even, healthy order of molecules. As a consequence, pathogens are removed from the tissue, nerve cells and even the DNA, as there is no room left between the molecules. In addition to successfully treating all kinds of pathogens, the Power Quick Zap also increases the bioenergy in a very short time (3 minutes), which can be proven through measurement in Bovis units. This means that the regeneration time of patients is shortened considerably. Reinfection becomes more difficult due to the body's strengthened energy.[113]

As I have explained, my personal experience using the device was also good. However, I heard from family and friends that the device was sometimes not well tolerated when the user was a heavy smoker

as they still had a high level of overacidification in the body.
Living conditions must therefore be optimised first. Only once harmful
things are avoided is it possible to heal slowly, and this also applies
to using this technique.
Martin Frischknecht has achieved good results in Africa, Asia and
Latin America with his different devices.[114] He was able to help people
there while also proving the effectiveness of his methods.

Investigations are currently being carried out by Professor Parlar at
Technische Universität München, the technical university in Munich.
According to Martin Frischknecht, the results so far are as follows:
1. The positive effect of the devices on human cells has been
proven.
2. After using the device for just 10 minutes the energy
potential of all test subjects increased measurably.

In summary, regularly using the devices can lead to complete detoxification
of the diseased cells. The results of the research are being pursued further
and being documented. Martin Frischknecht is also politically active in
Switzerland. As the lead representative of the Alpenparlament
organisation, he campaigned for the costs of complementary
medicine to be covered by statutory health insurance providers in
Switzerland in the same way as conventional medicine. In mid-2009,
the Swiss people voted for this to be made law with a majority of 67
percent. Since then, all costs for complementary medicine have been
covered by statutory health insurance in Switzerland. I fear that it
will be a long time before this is the case in Germany.


## 32. Trampolining

Trampolines provide a different kind of vibration. Soft, highly elastic
trampolines are particularly good for Parkinson's patients. It is not
about bouncing or jumping as with larger garden trampolines or those
used in sport, but simply about the vibration of the whole body. My

trampoline is 1.25m in diameter and is suitable for rooms of a normal height. This size is completely sufficient.

A key symptom of Parkinson's disease is dizziness and the associated balance problems that often lead to falls. In the beginning some form of support is often required when using a trampoline. This can be a handrail, a railing or someone who helps you to get on the trampoline and holds your hand during the exercises.

After initial tentativeness it is usually possible to do the vibration exercises alone after just a few days. You should then increase the amount of time gradually, which will increase general stability of posture and help counteract fear. In summary, a trampoline is an ideal method of preventing falls.

I would like to discuss the topic of lymph flow and detoxification again here. Vibration on the trampoline activates the sense of balance particularly well in the ear lymphs and strengthens the ability to balance. At the same time, it promotes the vitality of the brain. The supply of oxygen to the blood is increased considerably, while the vibration of the body cleanses the sinuses and removes harmful substances.[115] From my own experience I can say that vibration on the trampoline also supports the cleansing function of the intestine very well. Overall, the vibrations activate not only the main muscles but also the micromuscles in the whole body. Finally, with practice the ability to concentrate is also greatly improved.

## Other therapies

Therapies 33–42 discussed below are intended to supplement those above as I have not used all of them myself and have therefore either not been able to experience their effects or have not experienced them fully. This does not mean that they are any less valuable and it should not be taken as a negative judgement.

I want to make sure that the reader is aware of these therapies. I plan to collect more detailed information in the future and to report on the possibilities these natural methods have to offer, depending on how they progress.

I do not discuss conventional medical treatments, pharmacological therapy, Parkinson's patches or other methods such as implant therapy or the new stem cell therapy for Parkinson's disease that is currently still banned in Germany here. Instead I look at particular therapies used in natural medicine, complementary medicine and holistic medicine.
Chapter 43 describes the best therapy, early diagnosis.


## 33. Oxygen therapy

This therapy should be seen as a possible additional therapy, similar to physiotherapy in that it is not able to cure Parkinson's disease alone. However, the administration of oxygen brings a flood to our brain cells that brings freshness and concentration. I use a drop of liquid oxygen ($H_2O_2$), available from the pharmacy as 3% hydrogen peroxide, as standard every day. I use a dropper to put three to four drops into a quarter of a litre of good water such as Volvic or Evian in my water jug. I drink this enriched water over the course of the day.[116] The human brain needs at least 200 times more oxygen than the muscles of an athlete. Oxygen is ideally suited to regenerate the brain and the entire body, down to the smallest cell.
More extensive oxygen therapy can be recommended by a practitioner who will initially prescribe Parkinson's patients a full course of oxygen therapy once every six months. Later the periods between treatments can be extended considerably until they are only done once a year. Here the rule of 'less is more' applies. Talk to your practitioner for detailed advice. A good healthcare supply shop can also provide good advice.


## 34. Permanent acupuncture and other forms of acupuncture

I first learnt about the possibility of stimulating certain areas of the brain through permanent acupuncture around the ears in an article by neurologist Dr Ulrich Werth in the magazine *Fliege*.[117] There are over 200 different known reflex points in and around the ear that correspond to our organs. Acupuncture needles placed in the ear provide permanent stimulation to these reflex points that are recognised by the central nervous system and activate the powers of self-healing permanently. As a pleasant consequence, medications can usually be reduced.

Permanent acupuncture has its roots in traditional Chinese medicine (TCM). Here actual implants are placed in the energy channels to stimulate dopamine production. This decreases tremors, rigor, muscle stiffness and chronic pain and increases general everyday mobility.
Examples that demonstrate the effectiveness of acupuncture include the Bad Nauheim study by Professor Henneberg from the year 2002, the Saarlouis/Leipzig study from the same year and the Neumann study by the alternative practitioner Dr Claus-Peter Neumann from the year 2007. These studies show that the symptoms of rigor and tremor can be treated effectively with ear acupuncture in up to 70 percent of patients. They state costs of 800 to 1800 euros.[118] Most health insurance providers will not cover these costs.

Implant acupuncture is done with tiny needles that are inserted into the ear muscles. The puncture sites heal and are painless after two to three days. Research has shown that these implants often work for years. The effects become noticeable to the patient after around three to six weeks. The first neurological examination can be done after three months.

An alternative to these permanent implants made of pure titanium are semi-permanent needles. These are made of a degradable material and work for 15 to 20 months. Another Parkinson's sufferer told me about Dr Thomas Schockert's practice, where the methods of Dr Toshikatsu Yamamoto are used on Parkinson's patients. Here the therapists select acupuncture points on the forehead and temples. These methods have been used successfully in Japan since the 1960s.

The combined effects of acupuncture implants and an alkaline lifestyle with energy-rich food and cutting out nicotine and alcohol should not be underestimated, as adopting a natural diet and lifestyle increases the effects of this therapy.


## 35. Chelation therapy

Chelation therapy is an alternative to bypass operations and amputation for treating degenerative vascular disease. It is used to purify the blood vessels and remove heavy metals.[119]
Laid end to end the blood vessels in an adult human being – with a length of approximately 100,000 km – would stretch two and a half times around the Earth. Inner walls of the blood vessels that have been attacked are usually responsible for poor circulation. Poor circulation increases the risk of heart attacks, strokes and blockages such as plaques.

The blood vessels are purified with the mineral EDTA (ethylene diamine tetraacetic acid) as the main component of the chelation infusion. When adapted to the health of the patient, other substances used in complementary medicine that are selected according to the individual can also be added, such as coenzymes, carnitine or EPA 500. For Parkinson's patients coriander is often included, among other things.

Chelation therapy is often a very sensible alternative to bypass operations, cardiac catheterisation or amputations required due to peripheral artery disease in particular. The cleansing process usually requires several sessions of therapy and removes harmful heavy metals and other toxic substances. For Parkinson's patients this therapy is also used to remove heavy metals and other environmental toxins from the body, while expanding the blood vessels to improve circulation.

However, in my experience chelation therapy is not always as effective as desired in Parkinson's disease, an impression that many other sufferers have confirmed. As in some patients it is not possible to penetrate the blood-brain barrier, some crucial heavy metals remain in the brain. This happens, for example, when the heavy metals are embedded due to mutated fungi in the blood or other fungal infections, which is often the case in Parkinson's sufferers.


## 36. Indian healing plants

In my experience, healing plants used in Indian cultures are much more useful than chemical products in an approach that considers the mind, body and soul as one unit.

Harmine, a basic substance for modern psychoactive drugs, was developed from Indian healing plants such as the tropical ayahuasca. Natural harmine is a monoamine oxidase (MAO) inhibitor that prevents the break-down of neurotransmitters and works as an antidepressant. It also has a calming effect and reduces the break-down rate of serotonin in the body. Harmine has been proven to be effective against Parkinson's disease.[120]

Another healing plant is the (poisonous) angel's trumpet that can often be found in our gardens and in garden centres. With its large, dangling, trumpet-like flowers it is an ornamental plant that has been bred by horticulturalists and is a sister of the tree-height variety that grows in the tropics.

Another close relative is the datura, known for its thorny fruit. It is highly poisonous. Some of its poisons cause a state of intoxication. The famous Tonga tea – an infusion of datura made by the indigenous peoples of Columbia and Peru – slows down bodily function.[121] We also see this phenomenon in Parkinson's disease.

This therapy is similar to the homeopathic methods developed by Dr Hahnemann: treating like with like. The Native Americans use various plants to produce intoxicating drinks. Used for medical purposes, with the correct dosage and medical supervision, the effects can be highly beneficial for Parkinson's patients. Therapeutic doses of a few milligrammes have been used successfully in ophthalmology and in the treatment of Parkinson's disease.


## 37. Healing animal venoms

Many animal species that use venom to defend themselves effectively against foes can be found in nature. These venoms can often be beneficial for humans as, as Paracelsus said, the dose makes the poison.

Here are a few examples with regard to Alzheimer's and Parkinson's disease. The toxin secreted by the skin of the poison dart frog, found in Ecuador, was used by indigenous people in their deadly blowguns. This is poisonous to humans, but the poison dart frog has harmless relatives whose toxins can be used to treat Alzheimer's and Parkinson's disease effectively.[122]

It is a similar story with the venom of the green mamba. The dentrotoxins in the venom of these snakes enhances the release of the neurotransmitter acetylcholine (ACh). This substance can counteract Alzheimer's disease and possibly also Parkinson's disease.


## 38. Copper

In an article entitled *Kupfer für Alzheimer nach Prof. Dr. Pajonk* (copper treatment for Alzheimer's disease by Professor Pajonk), the author writes that many things indicate that a lack of copper in the brain is related to Alzheimer's disease. When administering additional copper, the progress of the disease has been observed to slow down or even stop in some patients.[123]

Veterinary medicine emphasises the high copper content of dandelion. Fresh dandelion is sold in markets in France from January to April, where it is known as pissenlit (literally 'bed wetter'). Dandelion is also often used in salads (called mesclun in French).
As its French name suggests, eating fresh dandelion is an effective way to flush out the kidneys. The bladder is cleansed and activated. After the blood has been cleansed by dandelion it can absorb oxygen better and transport it right to the smallest nerve cells in the brain.
Dandelion is mainly used to stimulate liver function and purify the liver. In particular, when removing amalgam from the teeth the liver should first be carefully prepared with a dandelion tincture four weeks beforehand.


## 39. Frankincense (Boswellia serrata)

A recommendation for Alzheimer's patients is to take frankincense H15, which can lead to mild improvement of the condition after just three weeks and considerable improvement after six weeks.[124] I heard about the possibilities of frankincense for treating illness rather late. Dr Ernst Schrott describes the treatment of individual cases of Alzheimer's disease, multiple sclerosis and other diseases in his book *Weihrauch* (frankincense).

I did not come across frankincense as medication in the form of H15; instead I used it in its original form, tree resin, as incense. By chance I discovered natural chunks of frankincense without any added colours or aromas in a monastery shop on Frauenchiemsee Island in Germany. I immediately wanted to try it out, so I bought a little and used it as incense at home. It should be used in moderation, but it clears the mind, makes it open for ideas and to enjoy life, and ensures a good general sense of wellbeing. The smoke gets into the fine structures inside the brain via the nose, where it can take effect. I used the frankincense once or twice a week and found it very successful. I have not tested frankincense capsules myself, as when I

read about them I had already been more or less cured.
Frankincense has been known for centuries in Ayurvedic medicine for
its smoke that disinfects and kills germs. It is certainly worth trying,
especially as so far no significant side effects have been identified.


## 40. Music and dance

In Parkinson's patients who are no longer able to walk even one
step in a straight line, dancing has been shown to improve
movement as if at the touch of a button. All of their movements
become smoother.[125]
Professor A. W. Harvey recommends slow pieces of music by Bach,
Vivaldi and Handel as they are particularly relaxing and stimulate
creativity.

The sound of music has a generally calming and revitalising effect.
Depression has decreased by 50 percent in some test subjects. Music
is a particularly ideal form of therapy for people with brain diseases
such as dementia and Parkinson's disease, as well as for people with
burn out and different forms of depression, particularly during the
darker months of the year. Music has been shown to activate the
limbic system. Listening to music can therefore be seen as a kind of
jogging for the brain.
This is particularly true of instrumental music. When listening to this
kind of music the density of the brain increases. The number of
synapses increases and the nerve cells become larger. In patients
who make music themselves, a whole range of processes are
triggered in the brain. For example, motor skills are improved, such
as the dexterity of the fingers when playing the piano or other
instruments.[126]
Dancing is a simple but effective way of implementing music in
controllable steps. It sounds easy, but in reality it is incredibly difficult
for Parkinson's patients, as the muscles do not always carry out the
orders sent by the brain.[127] Dancing is easier for patients who enjoyed

dancing before they became ill. Despite occasional difficulties in the beginning, dancing can be a wonderful therapy.


## 41. Paranormal surgery and trance medicine

Natural medicine has led me to many possibilities that can make a crucial contribution to healing. Sometimes even experienced alternative practitioners are not able to heal problems. It is therefore not enough to simply avoid chemical products. Even treatment with natural products does not always achieve the desired success.

One option here that can also be used by Parkinson's patients is to seek treatment through what is known as psychosurgery. For this treatment the patient is in a state of trance but is clearly conscious. This method has been used in Tibetan medicine for over 2700 years. Harmony with nature is the basis for this form of medicine, particularly for diseases that cannot be treated by any other method. These methods are complemented by dao yoga which is taught in different exercise steps. The background of this type of yoga, which cannot be compared with more widely known forms of yoga, strengthens and activates the powers of self-healing. The brain is usually only involved in self-healing at a rate of four percent in people with disease. The exercises allow this factor to be increased considerably.


## 42. Spiritual astrology and astromedicine

Astromedicine can be used to support treatment though natural medicine. It offers the patient the opportunity to recognise their own personal characteristics and behaviour patterns with the help of a therapist who is experienced in astrology. For example, blockages deep inside the person that prevent healing or cause disease in some way are recognised.
This information helps the sufferer to understand why they have the

disease. Here the guiding principle is that if you want to heal the body, you have to heal the soul first. This therapeutic approach is at the heart of the treatment of each patient, including those with Parkinson's disease. It is a search for causes on a mental level.

Astrology lists various diseases that are related to ascendants. It is often mental images from childhood that make people sick and affect the relationships, careers and lifestyles of those affected. Uncovering and recognising these images creates convincing and often surprising clarity with regard to the causes of disease and promotes healing as a consequence.


## 43. Early diagnosis – the best therapy

The best therapy is of course the prevention and early diagnosis of a disease. For this reason, I have made a list of various symptoms that could be early signs of Parkinson's disease. I created the following summary of Parkinson's symptoms to aid early diagnosis after having numerous discussions, collecting and processing the histories of the progression of the disease from sufferers, and considering the observations that I myself and other Parkinson's sufferers have made.

The initial symptoms are usually rather banal: simple changes in behaviour, hands occasionally shaking when drinking a cup of coffee, occasional forgetfulness ('Have I locked the front door?', 'Did I turn the oven off?'), knee problems occurring after walking or exercise, etc.

However, these things gradually occur more and more often and suddenly they are increasingly a part of everyday life. The initial symptoms take different forms in each patient of course, but my research and surveys have shown striking similarities. Those suffering from PSP (see part I, PSP) were mostly diagnosed with Parkinson's disease in the beginning. Some PSP patients have told me that they had had and been treated for Parkinson's disease for up to 12 years beforehand.

Here is a list of selected symptoms that may help identify Parkinson's disease at an early stage (symptoms marked with * were mentioned by at least 60 percent of those asked):

constant tiredness*
loss of sense of smell*
problems concentrating; often forgetting names and events ('What did I just say?') *
walk changes, becomes slower, appears stiffer*
steps become smaller and/or shuffling*
when walking pressure is on the outsides of the feet
withdrawal ('I just want to be left in peace')*
veering to the left or to the right when walking*
swaying when walking, as if drunk
circulation problems when standing still
no longer being able to get dressed independently*
weight loss
loss of interest; feeling insecure, distrusting*
difficulty controlling arm movements
difficulty controlling movements in general*
sudden arm or leg movements, especially at night*
shaking hands, tremor and resting tremor*
jerky movements*
voice becomes quiet and hoarse, voice husky
dizziness*
horrible dreams with lots of blood and body parts despite never having actually seen such images in war or in an accident
work and career no longer important, more difficult*
extreme itching on the edge of either or both hands
frequent and constant sneezing, 10 to 20 times in a row
things often fall out of your hand
breaking out in sweat at night; pillow and covers are wet
fear, especially fear of falling, fear of being in a wheel chair, fear of everyday life*
fear/breaking out in sweat when the telephone rings*
dry mouth*
handwriting changes, becoming smaller and later scrawled and

illegible
increased yawning at any time of day, also when outside
buzzing and whistling noises in one or both ears*
eyes burn, tear fluid feels like it burns
facial expressions become more immobile, almost like a mask
noticeably less resilient*
desire to be in the sun and in nature*
fear at night, e.g. fear of seeing ghosts
increasingly frequent back pain*
pain in the legs
cramp in the feet
back becomes more and more hunched*
fear when walking on steep paths, roads, wheelchair ramps
problems swallowing; particularly at night saliva accumulates due to
lack of swallowing reflex, resulting in coughing*
mental block, particularly after being in a position of great
responsibility for many years*
difficulty reading; no longer understanding all of what you read
fear of reading aloud due to articulation worsening
uncertainty in discussions; losing the thread of the conversation*
fear of crowds*
mental anguish; wanting to organise things but no longer being able
to*
extreme slowness results in anger and feelings of helplessness*
not knowing what is going on; forgetting what you wanted to do*
feeling insecure when driving, particularly when there are
construction works, when it is raining or at night
no longer being able to drive at all
balance problems*
increased emotional sensitivity, e.g. crying or feeling sad easily*
sudden falls*
frequently banging your head
not being able to do two things at once, e.g. turning around while
walking
not wanting to take medication

oversensitivity
strong itching around the calves or ankles
strong itching around the anus
bleeding on the calves, dark/viscous (visible in the case of minor
wounds)*, ulcer
whole body not functioning normally
everything feels confused*
alternating diarrhoea, constipation and hard stool*
history of rheumatic diseases, e.g. in childhood
sudden reluctance to use toxins, e.g. weed killer, mosquito spray*
listlessness, e.g. just wanting to sit down*
saliva accumulates in the mouth when talking*
spots or scabs behind the earlobes
feet hurt yet feel increasingly less pain as a result of external
influences, e.g. pricking the skin
no longer feeling the tuning fork in doctors' tests*
controlled grasping of objects becomes more difficult

When I first became ill I wrote around eight of these symptoms down
on a piece of paper so that I could discuss them with my doctor. I
would not have been able to remember them during my appointment
otherwise. Yet the doctor said to me, 'You should never show my
colleagues anything like that. Otherwise be prepared for them to
consider you a hypochondriac.' I think the doctor meant well.
Unfortunately, he did not know what to do with my observations. He
only wrote two of the symptoms down in his notes: the tremor and the
fears.

If you notice five or more of the symptoms listed above for an
extended period of time, this should be an alarm signal. Even if you
are not yet sure whether it is Parkinson's disease, you must recognise
that they are an indication of a disease of some kind. This should be
clear at that point.

In my experience and according to my extensive research, almost all lifestyle diseases, including Parkinson's disease, Alzheimer's disease and multiple sclerosis, are largely due to the same causes: overacidification, toxification due to heavy metals and medications, the expansion of fungi, leeches, worms and similar in the blood and intestine, and the effects of earth radiation, water veins and electro smog.

This should be reason enough to start living consciously and to immediately begin practicing an alkaline lifestyle, have your blood analysed using dark field microscopy, and to select the right therapies from the suggestions above and discuss them with a specialist who you trust.

You should travel, get to know other cities and places, learn languages, dance, play music or paint if you feel that you want to. It provides distraction and keeps the brain active. Any kind of activity is what you need, instead of resignation. Ignore the popular scary diagnoses such as 'You'll have to live with this from now on', 'Parkinson's is an incurable disease' or 'You should be prepared to be in a wheelchair in five years.'

In my experience, chemical medications with their harmful side effects should be the last resort.

With this statement I am turning the conventional approach to Parkinson' disease on its head: usually after unsuccessful treatment with conventional medicine patients who are deemed incurable are finally 'given permission' by their doctor to try natural medicine.

If this leads to improvement then it is not a miracle or a placebo effect. Such an event can only be explained by the changes in the body caused by a lifestyle rich in vitamins and minerals – moving away from chemicals and towards nature.

In Antiquity, Socrates explained this as follows: It is not because things are difficult that we do not dare, it is because we do not dare that things are difficult.

I therefore plead for change. Lead a healthy life through to old age – and start in time or, better yet, start early. It should be worth the effort for you. Investigate the possibilities of natural medicine with regard to healing. Be aware that chemical medications only treat the symptoms of disease.

In my experience, medications only prolong disease. The side effects cause more diseases, which in turn require more medications, which have more side effects, and so on and so on. It is like a hamster wheel; you can never get out.

You control your health. To do this what you need to start with is a clear head. Always be critical and confident when dealing with the people who are treating you. It does not matter what their specialism is, as for some of them it is your health that is important while for some of them it is money, and for some it is both.

By the way, whenever you are required to make a decision about your heath there is always enough time for you to sleep on it for at least a day or two. Never let your doctor or alternative practitioner pressure you.

# Part III
# Health as a foundation

# The first steps

These suggestions are intended to help you to understand and recognise the main toxins and things that make us ill that are present in our everyday lives. Based on my experience, the list of products and manufacturing practices that can cause illness that you will find below is only the tip of the iceberg.

The first sensible measures

Particularly important: you must give up alcohol, tobacco and drugs. These dangerous and poisonous substances make it impossible to heal.

Take off all metals, watches and rings as they can block the flow of energy through the meridians, particularly if disease is present. You should identify all objects and habits that cause disease and ban them from your life. Otherwise they can lead to energy blockages in the immune regulation.

The individual points in the following lists are all unacceptable in my opinion. However, the degree of harmfulness varies greatly. Some of them are unlikely to have serious consequences if used or done once, while others can cause irreparable damage in the body. I have only listed some of the most important examples here. Please consult the books and magazines mentioned for more detailed information.

Habits that can cause disease

*Reheated meals* contain very few natural vitamins after being reheated and the minerals lose their beneficial effects.[1]

*Ready meals, frozen food and packet soups* are as lacking in nutritional value as reheated food.

*Aluminium foil:* baked goods and other foods that are wrapped or heated in aluminium foil[2, 3, 4]

Food that is packaged in aluminium foil

Aluminium trays

Scraping off or licking aluminium lids (e.g. on yoghurt pots)

Packaging that is coated with aluminium on the inside and/or aluminium packaging in general

From a medical point of view, aluminium is extremely harmful to the brain.

*Microwave:* destroys the nutrients[5, 6]

*Ready meals or coffee* that are put into Styrofoam containers when hot. This causes styrene to be released.

*Glutamate,* a flavour enhancer in soups and ready meals[7, 8]

*Gluten:* for people who react sensitively to it

*Conserves* of all kinds that contain chemical preservatives

*Chemical preservatives*[9]

*Pasteurised food:* the vitamins and minerals in them no longer have their full effect.

*Fizzy drinks:* cola and other fizzy drinks contain too much industrial sugar and phosphoric acid.

*Diet drinks* of all kinds weaken the bones.

*Diet foods* cause weight gain; they often cause people to want more.[10]

*Sweeteners:* chemical sweeteners such as aspartame are extremely harmful in the long term.[11]

*Coffee whiteners:* if chemical

*White sugar:* industrial crystalline sugar is harmful, not just because of nanoparticles.[12–15]

*White flour:* no nutritional value

*Milk products with less than 2 percent fat:* the minerals cannot be absorbed by the body.[16, 17, 18]
Products with *harmful E numbers* and preservatives[19]
*Margarine*: too much harmful hydrogenated fat
*Mouldy food:* including food that has only just begun to go mouldy, such as cheese, bread, jam, tomatoes or oranges[20]
*Citric acid:* manufactured chemically from the fungus Aspergillus nigra that allows aluminium to penetrate the blood-brain barrier and become deposited in the brain[21]
*Heavy metals:* e.g. in mushrooms, tuna and other foods (it is ok to eat them occasionally as these products also contain important minerals)[22, 23]
*Vaccines:* in Germany many vaccines contain harmful substances such as thiomersal (mercury) and formaldehyde.[24, 25, 26]
*Lead pipes* in the domestic water supply (often still found in old buildings)[27, 28]
*Tattoos, permanent make-up and piercings* are very harmful due to the heavy metals or other metals in them; abrasion, saliva or sweat can release them, allowing them into the body.
*Amalgam* used in dental filling[29, 30]
*Cholesterol*[31]
*Fried food* (acrylamide) if produced industrially; home-made chips made of organic potatoes, on the other hand, are not a problem
All *crisps* due, for example, to the hydrogenated fat and monosodium glutamate (MSG) which can also be contained in organic crisps[32]
*Formaldehyde*: domestic toxins in upholstery, plastic flooring, etc.[33]
*Neurotoxins:* chemical toxins that harm the nerves such as ethanol, formalin, arsenic, and many more
*Propyl alcohol:* also called propanol or isopropanol; found in cosmetics, cereals, cornflakes and much more[34]
*PCB – polychlorinated biphenyl:* carcinogenic chemical compound of chlorine found in varnishes, sealants, etc.; number one immune killer[35]

---

*Fluorine:* toothpaste, added to things in kindergartens as well as to water (check ingredients)[36, 37]
*Chlorine:* in the home, check water values stated by water supplier[38]
*Vinegar:* e.g. for salads; tip: use lemon for acidity, this is suitable for an alkaline lifestyle
*Salt:* exceptions: fleur de sel and Himalayan salt
*Carbonated water:* ideally avoid altogether[39, 40]
*Genetically modified food:* consequences unknown, better to avoid
*Processed meats*: not recommended due to industrial additives such as phosphates and nitrates[41]
*Meat:* only eat occasionally; exceptions can be made for organic meat if you trust the butcher who supplies it
*Isopropyl alcohol:* mouth wash, shampoos, disinfectant, etc.
*Silicon:* found in creams and soaps
*Deodorants* contain fine traces of aluminium – even deodorant stones available from organic shops
*Lotions* contain softening agents
*Softening agents* are found all around the home, for example in industrial soaps or washing up liquid
*Chemical domestic cleaning products* contain toxins[42]
*Weed killer* and other environmental toxins
*Pesticides:* high amount of heavy metals
*Insecticides*
*Moth balls*
*Mosquito spray*
*Waterproofing products*
*Wood protector*[43, 44, 45]
*Electro smog*
*Mobile communications radiation*
*Computer radiation*
*Electrical power line radiation*
*Mobile phone radiation*[46, 47, 48]
*Biopharmaceuticals* (medications produced using genetic engineering)

*Earth radiation* caused by water veins, faults or Curry grids (or Hartmann grids) is often a cause of Parkinson's disease. The harmful influences vary in severity and should be determined by a specialist.[49, 50]

Here are a few more proven immune killers, taken from an article in the September 2009 issue of *Welt der Wunder* magazine entitled 'Die Terroristen in unserem Essen: Billig, lecker, tödlich – Millionen sterben an Industriefood'[51] (the terrorists in our food: cheap, tasty, deadly – millions die from industrial food).

The phosphoric acid found in many types of cola weakens the bones. Cola drinkers have a significantly lower bone density. This has been observed in women especially. Phosphoric acid is used to balance out the taste of the excessively high sugar content.

Soft foods cause weight gain. For this reason, avoid soft foods such as sliced bread, cake, doughnuts, creams, etc. People who choose harder food that must be chewed thoroughly have a smaller waistline.

Eating more than 500g of red meat per week can cause bowel cancer. Heme molecules give meats its red colour. They take oxygen from the blood to transfer it to the muscles which allows greater endurance. When we eat red meat these heme molecules get into our bowel and damage the bowel walls.

Ham, bacon and salami cause cancer in two ways. In addition to heme molecules, nitrates are added to processed meats to make them last longer. The meat retains its nice deep-red colour, making it look more appetising. These nitrates can cause tumours in the digestive system. Watch out for E249 and E250!

Iced coffee is often blamed for tumours as it is usually prepared with milk, cream and sugar syrup. This causes an energy surplus which is stored as fat. For this reason, tumour researchers warn people about these drinks.

Stay away from crisps! Crisps made from reformed potatoes are made of a flavourless mixture of potatoes, wheat and corn. The flavour comes from salt and monosodium glutamate (MSG). In high doses this becomes a neurotoxin that is even able to pass through the blood-brain barrier, making us permanently hungry for this toxin. Muesli bars make us hungry. The main ingredient is a sugar substitute, corn syrup. The food industry uses this to get us to consume more and more of it. This is caused by free fructose, a form of fructose which can only be broken own in the liver. Too much of it puts strain on the liver, meaning that it can no longer fulfil the tasks that it is actually intended to do. Some medical experts rightly warn people against consuming too many products that contain corn syrup. Cornflakes have an incredibly high sugar content. This is well known. However, large quantities of salt are required so that the consumer does not notice the sugar. The taste of the salt is hidden by the taste of the sugar. This is particularly bad for children as they can only tolerate small amounts of salt. This means that they already get an overdose of salt at breakfast, the consequence of which is that the body retains more fluid and the blood pressure rises. These children are the cardiac patients of tomorrow.

Energy drinks remove water from the body in the intestine. The liquid, coupled with caffeine and sugar (cheap corn syrup) is supposed to increase energy reserves. For the body to process this mixture the intestine has to remove water from the body. Drinking these drinks therefore leads to negative effects on hydration.
Jelly is an entirely artificial food. The most important colouring in green jelly is quinoline yellow, sometimes known simply as E104. It is suspected to cause cancer and allergies, as well as hyperactivity similar to ADHD in children, and to be responsible for lower IQs. Researchers consider it as harmful as lead. Quinoline yellow is banned in the United Kingdom.
Gummy bears and baked goods often contain the flavour enhancer maltol. This substance causes the body's cells to absorb more aluminium, which acts as a neurotoxin and causes certain types of dementia such as Alzheimer's disease, as well as Parkinson's disease. Maltol is difficult to spot on packaging because it is often disguised as caramel or caramel extract. Maltol is most easily identified as an

ingredient by its E number, E636.
In Germany, marzipan usually contains the additive butylated
hydroxyanisole (BHA) as a preservative. BHA is banned in Austria and
its use is restricted in the USA. This substance is not water soluble
and can therefore not be removed from the body and accumulates in
fat tissue. It is responsible for rashes and various allergies, and can
even affect foetuses in the womb. Watch out for BHA or E320!
Sugar-coated chocolate drops are dangerous, especially the blue ones.
They can cause rashes, allergies and, in the worst case, fatal shock.
The colouring known as Patent Blue V or E131 is responsible. This
colouring is banned in Norway, Australia and the USA.

... and that is just the tip of the iceberg when it comes to the harmful
substances in industrial food. These are just a few examples.
The risks described above are particularly dangerous because they
are not all mentioned in the list of E numbers. Why not?
Please refer to a list of E numbers when you are shopping to ensure at
least some safety. Be critical of the promises advertised on packaging.
After all, your health is at stake!

*Take the first step in faith.*
*You don't have to see the whole staircase,*
*just take the first step.*
(Martin Luther King Jr.)

Trust is the first step and the first requirement for change!
Here I would like to make it clear again that I am a layman when it
comes to medicine and all of the information in this book, and in
particular in the work sheets on the following pages, is based solely
on my personal experience. I am therefore obliged to state the
following: in the case of serious illness, you must consult your doctor
or alternative practitioner. I would also like to refer to the liability
disclaimer at the beginning of the book.

Observations of myself and other Parkinson's patients have led me to recognise a surprisingly simple basic structure. Essentially, all those who say that Parkinson's disease is due to overacidification are right. Those who say that Parkinson's disease is a disease of the liver are right. And those who say that Parkinson's disease is caused by severe heavy metal toxification, fungi, leeches, bacteria, stress, fear, etc., etc., etc. are right. Of course, the influence of each of these causative factors differs greatly in each case. Essentially, however, the cause is always a combination of these factors. To put it another way, in my opinion, one of the harmful factors listed above is never the sole cause of Parkinson's disease. For this reason, I can never recommend using just one of the therapies described in part II of this book. Parkinson's disease and many other lifestyle diseases should be viewed as complex puzzles or mosaics in which each cause of illness plays a different role in the overall picture. However, we can also recognise how easily we can remove the causes of disease through natural methods if it is recognised at an early stage. If used consistently, over time the various therapies selected can lead to an entirely new picture of comprehensive health and happiness. Just as we have made our bodies sick with decades of a poor lifestyle, we can usually consciously correct this with healthy therapies in just a few years.

## Work sheet 1
## Self-observation

Recognising the causes of the disease

In order to recognise Parkinson's disease you must of course recognise the possible causes. I have therefore made a list of ten groups of causes based on my experience. Please take your time to consider them before moving on to work sheet 2.

1. Soul/psyche
   - mental block
   - unprocessed experiences from childhood
   - traumatic situations experienced by mother during
     pregnancy

2. Body
   - diseases of organs, such as liver diseases
   - lymphatic diseases, particularly diseases of
     the lymph nodes in the head
   - diseases of the pancreas, lungs, spleen, intestine, gallbladder,
     kidneys, small intestine, large intestine, skin, etc.
   - lack of vitamins and minerals

3. Impurities and infections
   - intestinal fungi, viruses, bacteria, leeches, Lyme disease,
     mutated fungi/camouflaged candida or similar in the
     blood, accumulations of the same in the brain, etc.

4. Overacidification
   - overacidification of all affected organs such as the liver, kidney,
     skin, blood, etc.

5. Toxification
   - side effects of medications
   - environmental toxins
   - heavy metals
   - amalgam, mercury, palladium and similar
   - insecticides, pesticides, wood protector
   - softening agents in cosmetics and

plastics
- aluminium, manganese and lead
- carbon monoxide
- diesel particles
- toxins from food
- domestic toxins, formaldehyde and more
- vaccinations
- medications, in particular antipsychotics or calcium channel blockers

6. Lifestyle
- poor nutrition
- harmful foods, glutamate, aspartame, etc.
- lemonade, processed meats, phosphates, etc.
- harmful lifestyle, e.g. hectic lifestyle, stress, cigarettes
- alcohol
- fast food
- junk food

7. Brain/mind
- multiple-system atrophy = degeneration of the structures and systems of the central nervous system (CNS) due to, for example:
- stroke
- meningitis
- brain tumour
- bleeding in the brain in the substantia nigra
- drug consumption
- injections of pethidine analogues
- Creutzfeldt–Jakob disease
- lack of minerals
- lack of vitamins
- overacidification
- heavy metals (e.g. amalgam)

- damaged blood terrain
- borrelia, trichomonads, Mucor mucedo, etc.

8. ADD/ADHD
- in childhood, for example, and consuming medications from an early age as a result

9. Consequences of accidents
- falls or knocks, impacts on the head, etc.
- even seemingly simple falls where the spine was damaged which may have happened several years before
- sports injuries, risks from sport, etc.

10. Environment
- geopathic features
- water veins
- earth radiation
- Hartmann grids, etc.
- electro smog,
- magnetic fields
- radio masts
- noise pollution, motorways, airports, cities, etc.
- light pollution in cities

11. Your own suspicions and findings

..........................................................................
..........................................................................

When were you explicitly diagnosed with Parkinson's disease?

..........................................................................

What did the doctor determine as the cause (not symptoms)?

..........................................................................

If unknown, make sure you ask!

Medications you are taking:
since when?
daily dosage:

..........................................................................
..........................................................................
..........................................................................

Have you read all of the information leaflets carefully and discussed them
with your doctor?
yes/no

# Work sheet 2
# Your own findings

(reproduction and copying not permitted)

The following list of problems and symptoms is based on my own experience of Parkinson's disease. Please go through it carefully point by point. Discuss the list with a doctor, alternative practitioner or other professional who you trust. Considering your medical history in advanced will help you and the person treating you when looking for advice; it will give you security and reassure you that you have not forgotten to mention anything. It will also provide the person treating you with information that they need to determine exactly what has happened to you and which areas of the body need to be monitored and which need to be treated.

Before you start, please pause for a minute to think. Think in love and thanks of the people who help you every day in some way. Think of the 'man upstairs' and ask him for help healing. If you do not believe in God think very consciously about the healing of your body and your mind. Now start the work sheet, feeling calm and balanced.

Based on my experience, the points marked * to *** are particularly significant in Parkinson's disease.

## General

| | |
|---|---|
| Do you show typical signs of the early stages of Parkinson's disease?<br>(see chapter on early diagnosis)<br> If yes, which? | |
| Do you have any allergies?<br>If yes, which? | |
| What are your favourite foods? | |
| How much do you drink per day? (in litres)?:<br>Water***　　　　　　　Fizzy drinks<br>Tea***　　　　　　　　Coffee<br>Alkaline herbal tea***　　Fresh vegetable juice***<br>Alkaline fruit tea　　　　Fresh fruit juice***<br>Wine　　　　　　　　　Beer<br>Milk | |
| Left-handed or right-handed? | right/left |
| Do you parents have any significant illnesses? | |
| Father's illnesses: | |
| Mother's illnesses: | |
| Children: | yes/no |
| | son(s)　　　　daughter(s) |
| Illnesses diagnosed in children (not including childhood illnesses): | |

| | |
|---|---|
| Illnesses diagnosed in grandchildren (not including childhood illnesses): | |
| Do you sleep through the night? | yes/no |
| Dreams at night about: | daily life    stress    horror    violence |
| Dreams in quiet moments during the day: | happiness    worry    horror    violence |
| Thoughts focus on: | family    neighbours    friends<br>holiday    accident    death |
| Star sign:* | |
| Date of birth: | |
| Hour and minute of birth: | |
| Urine:* | colour:***<br>pH value: 4 a.m.: …… 7 a.m.:……… |
| Bowel movements** | regular: yes/no<br>in 24 hours: ………… times |
| Faecal residue floating in the toilet:*** | yes/no |
| Diarrhoea: | rarely    always    varies |
| Constipation: | rarely    always    varies |
| Problems in urogenital area: | yes/no |
| Loss of sense of smell:*** | yes/no<br>if yes, since when? ………… |
| Loss of sense of taste: | yes/no<br>if yes, since when? ………… |

| | |
|---|---|
| Problems swallowing:*** | yes/no<br>if yes, since when?...............<br>at night***    during the day |
| Metals in the blood:*** | yes/no |
| Overacidification:*** | yes/no |
| Heart problems:* | yes/no |
| Blood pressure:* | value: ............ |
| Blood sugar:* | value:............ |
| Cholesterol:* | value: ............ |
| Homocysteine:*** | value from last blood test: ...... |
| Biliary colic:*** | yes/no<br>if yes, when? ......<br>surgery when? ...... |
| Renal colic:** | yes/no<br>if yes, when?......<br>surgery when?...... |
| Skin:* | smooth<br>cracked/chapped<br>wounds/eczema |
| Uncontrolled salivation *** | yes/no<br>if yes:<br>when speaking        at night |
| Hallucinations:** | yes/no |
| Hunched back:* | yes/no |
| Universal energy pulse diagnosis*** | yes/no<br>if yes: result:............ |
| Ayurveda pulse diagnosis:*** | yes/no<br>if yes: result:............ |
| Visible acids/toxin deposits on the body:*** | yes/no<br>if yes: knee   wrist   ankle   feet<br>other:................... |

## Problems

| | |
|---|---|
| Head:*** I suddenly keep hitting my head. | yes/no |
| Central nervous system:*** I fall suddenly. | yes/no |
| Can no longer control arm and leg movements | arms: yes/no <br> legs: yes/no <br> if yes: at night   during the day <br> how often? ………… |
| Thought blockage:*** I lose track of things. | yes/no |
| Brain activity:*** I zone out when reading, making calculations, drawing. | yes/no |
| Handwriting:*** | getting smaller <br> signature scrawled/illegible |
| Concentration:*** | |
| Memory loss concerning: | names   facts   yesterday <br> next appointment <br> other: ……………………… |
| Thoughts:*** | happiness   gloom   depression |
| Mental block:*** | yes/no <br> if yes, when? ………………… |
| Confusion:*** What was it that I wanted? | yes/no |
| Dementia:*** | yes/no <br> if yes, since when?……………… |

| | |
|---|---|
| Compulsions:*** <br> Have I turned everything off; have I left everything where it should be? | yes/no |
| Fear:*** | of crowds: yes/no <br> of the telephone: yes/no <br> when paths are steep: yes/no <br> when reading aloud: yes/no <br> of falling: yes/no <br> of being in wheelchair: yes/no <br> of the future: yes/no <br> of no longer being strong: yes/no |
| Withdrawal: <br> I just want to be left in peace. | yes/no |
| Emotions:*** | crying    moaning <br> uncontrolled temper |
| Thoughts: <br> I have been cast aside. <br> It will not get better. | yes/no |
| Personal motivation: <br> I want to know now. <br> I am still needed. | yes/no |
| Motivation:*** | none    rarely    often    always |
| Work: | important/unimportant |
| Desire for:*** | quiet    peace <br> sun    nature |
| Restlessness:*** | yes/no <br> if yes: <br> internal        visible |

| | |
|---|---|
| Uncertainty:** <br> Everything makes me uncertain; people, driving | yes/no |
| Voice:*** | husky   hoarse   becoming quieter |
| Face:*** | lively expression     mask-like <br> indifferent expression <br> shiny/greasy |
| Eyes:** | burning: yes/no <br> vision** …………% |
| Deposits in the corners of the eyes: | yes/no |
| Iris diagnosis:*** | yes/no <br> if yes, when? …………… <br> result: ……………… |
| Ears:* | pressure: yes/no <br> ringing: yes/no <br> if yes: right/left |
| Earwax: | yes/no <br> if yes, how often? …… <br> colour: …………… |
| Dizziness:* | yes/no <br> if yes: <br> sometimes***     constantly |
| Balance problems:*** | yes/no <br> if yes: <br> indoors   outdoors |
| Facial diagnosis:*** | yes/no <br> if yes: result:……………… |
| Hair: | hair loss: yes/no <br> going bald: yes/no |

| Nose:* | running |
|---|---|
| | constant sneezing up to … times |
| Sinuses***/cranial cavity: | inflammation: yes/no |
| | deposits: yes/no |
| Sinuses:*** | problems: yes/no |
| | if yes, where?......... |
| | surgery when? ......... |
| Mouth: ** | smell: yes/no |
| Oral mucosa: | inflammation: yes/no |
| Saliva: *** | building up in mouth: yes/no |
| | if yes: runny   thick |
| Yawning: *** | rarely   often   also outdoors |
| Speech: *** | clear   unclear   varies |
| Problems swallowing: *** | yes/no |
| | if yes: |
| | at night     during the day |
| | rarely        always |
| Tongue:*** | normal   coating   colour: ...... |
| Teeth*** | amalgam fillings |
| | bridges/crowns |
| (Dead) teeth with root canal:*** | yes/no |
| Prosthetics: | yes/no |
| Misaligned jaw: | yes/no |
| | if yes: right/left |
| Maxillary sinus: *** | problems: yes/no |
| | if yes, where? .............. |
| | surgery when?......... |

| Test: | |
|---|---|
| Write the time in figures: ** | e.g. 1.50 p.m. |
| Read a short newspaper article aloud: | quick   faltering<br>no longer possible |
| Brain training: ** | 175 ÷ 35 = …<br>Seconds taken: ……… |
| Urination: | when?……<br>stinging: yes/no<br>trickling: yes/no |
| Sweating:* | during the day***<br>at night***<br>smell:……………… |
| Itching:* | anus: yes/no<br>side of hand: yes/no<br>if yes: right/left<br>calves: yes/no<br>if yes: right/left |
| Stabbing pain:* | yes/no<br>if yes, where? ……………… |
| Tingling:* | yes/no<br>if yes, where? ……………… |
| Hands shaking:*** | yes/no<br>if yes:<br>right/left   always   rarely |
| Resting tremor: | yes/no<br>if yes: shakes per minute:…… |

| Atlas correction:*** | yes/no<br>if yes, when? ..................... |
|---|---|
| Arms: | arthrosis: yes/no<br>rigidity: yes/no<br>if yes: right/left |
| Movements no longer controlled: | yes/no |
| If movement is limited: | slower    stiffer |
| If pain: | where?......... |
| Elbows: | epicondylitis: yes/no<br>arthrosis: yes/no<br>if yes: right/left |
| Hands: | gout: yes/no<br>arthrosis: yes/no<br>if yes: right/left |
| Carpal tunnel syndrome: | yes/no<br>if yes, since when?<br>right/left<br>surgery when? |
| Back: *** | straight        increasingly bent<br>frequent pain |
| Cervical spine: *** | C problems: ........... yes/no<br>if yes, surgery when?......... |
| Thoracic spine:*** | T problems: ........... yes/no<br>if yes, surgery when?......... |
| Lumbar spine:*** | L problems: ........... yes/no<br>if yes, surgery when?......... |

| | |
|---|---|
| Slipped disc:*** | yes/no<br>if yes: cervical spine ………<br>thoracic spin ………<br>lumbar spine ……… |
| Pelvis:* | pelvic obliquity: yes/no<br>if yes: right/left |
| Hips:* | problems: yes/no<br>if yes: right/left<br>surgery when?……… |
| Muscles*** | |
| Legs:* | one leg shorter: yes/no<br>if yes: …… mm |
| Shoes worn: | yes/no<br>if yes: right/left |
| Gait: *** | wobbly<br>veering to the left<br>veering to the right |
| Changes in gait: | yes/no<br>if yes: slower   stiffer<br>no longer controllable<br>smaller steps |
| Able to walk heel first: | yes/no |
| Able to walk on tiptoes: | yes/no |
| Walking on the inside of the foot: | yes/no |
| Walking on the outside of the foot:*** | yes/no<br>if yes: right/left |
| Knee problems: | yes/no<br>if yes: right/left<br>surgery when?…… |

| | |
|---|---|
| Feet: | problems: yes/no if yes: right/left<br>surgery when?...... |
| Endocrine glands | |
| Pituitary gland:*** | problems: yes/no<br>if yes, since when? ...... |
| Pineal gland:*** | problems: yes/no<br>if yes, since when? ...... |
| Thyroid gland:*** | problems: yes/no<br>if yes, since when? ...... |
| Thymus:*** | problems: yes/no<br>if yes, since when? ...... |
| Pancreas:*** | problems: yes/no<br>if yes, since when? ...... |
| Gonads: | problems: yes/no<br>if yes, since when? ...... |
| Specific organs | |
| Lungs: | problems: yes/no<br>pulmonary function test: yes/no<br>surgery ............ |
| Kidneys:*** | problems: yes/no<br>if yes: right/left<br>surgery ............ |
| Adrenal glands: | problems: yes/no<br>if yes: right/left<br>surgery ............ |
| Liver:*** | problems: yes/no<br>if yes<br>surgery ............ |

| Gall bladder:*** | problems: yes/no<br>if yes:<br>surgery ............ |
|---|---|
| Spleen:*** | problems: yes/no<br>if yes:<br>surgery ............ |
| Stomach:*** | problems: yes/no<br>if yes:<br>surgery ............ |
| Small intestine:** | problems: yes/no<br>if yes:<br>surgery ............ |
| Large intestine:** | problems: yes/no<br>if yes:<br>surgery ............ |
| Duodenum: | problems: yes/no<br>if yes:<br>surgery ............ |
| Bladder:** | problems: yes/no<br>if yes:<br>surgery ............ |
| Prostate:** | problems: yes/no<br>if yes:<br>surgery ............ |
| Genitals: | problems: yes/no<br>if yes:<br>surgery ............ |
| Anus:* | problems: yes/no<br>if yes: bleeding    itching |

| **Other events/problems/diseases** | |
|---|---|
| ADD/ADHD: | yes/no |
| Consequences of accident(s): | yes/no<br>if yes, which? ..................... |
| Strokes: | yes/no |
| Infections: | yes/no<br>if yes, which? ..................... |
| Heart attack: | yes/no<br>if yes, which? ..................... |
| Transplants: | yes/no<br>if yes, which? .....................<br>when? ......... |
| Rheumatic diseases: | yes/no<br>if yes, which? ..................... |
| Amputations: | yes/no<br>if yes, which? ..................... |
| Cancer: | yes/no<br>if yes, which? ..................... |
| Eye diseases: | yes/no<br>if yes, which? ..................... |
| Diabetes: | yes/no<br>if yes, which? ..................... |
| Other: | yes/no<br>if yes, which?..................... |
| Other questions about and explanations for the problems above: | |

## Blood tests

There are two essentially two ways to identify diseases in the blood.
Conventional blood tests determine important parameters such as
cholesterol, blood sugar, blood pressure, uric acid and homocysteine.
Important aspects that are identified by examining the blood through
dark field microscopy are the Parkinson's factor, overacidification,
heavy metal toxification, candida and other fungi, bacteria, acids,
oxygen content, Lyme disease, worms, leeches, the concentration of
symbionts, etc. Some of the most revealing information here is the C
values (C stands for camouflaged) for trichomonads and candida
fungi. Ekkehard Scheller discovered these toxins through his research
in 1995.[52]
Both types of tests should be carried out as the values complement
each other well.


## Which treatments and/or examinations have you had so far?

Mark your answers as follows:
D (by a doctor)
A (alternative practitioner)
O (on your own)

| Cortisone treatments in the last 5 years: | yes/no<br>if yes: injections   tablets<br>cream | D<br>A<br>O |
|---|---|---|
| Antibiotic treatments in the last 5 years: | yes/no<br>if yes: injections   tablets<br>cream | |
| Colon cleansing in the last 5 years: | yes/no<br>if yes, when? ........... | |
| Psychotherapy: | yes/no<br>if yes, since when?<br>..................... | |
| Energy transfer: | yes/no<br>if yes: yourself<br>by other people | |
| Physiotherapy: | yes/no<br>if yes, which area? ...........<br>per week: ........... | |
| Occupational therapy: | yes/no<br>if yes, since when? ...........<br>per week: ........... | |
| Feldenkrais therapy: | yes/no<br>if yes, since when?........... per week: ........... | |
| Speech therapy: | yes/no<br>if yes, since when? ...........<br>per week: ........... | |
| Yoga: | yes/no<br>if yes, since when? .........<br>per week: ........... | |

| | | |
|---|---|---|
| Water aerobics: | yes/no<br>if yes, since when?………… per<br>week: ………… | |
| Acupuncture: | yes/no<br>if yes, since when? …………<br>per week: ………… | |
| Acupressure: | yes/no<br>if yes, since when? …………<br>per week: ………… | |
| Permanent acupuncture: | yes/no<br>if yes, since when? …………<br>area: …………… | |
| Meridian therapy: | yes/no   if yes, which area?<br>………………………….<br>no. sessions so far: …… | |
| Ayurvedic detoxification: | yes/no<br>if yes, when? …………<br>where? ……………… | |
| Dark field microscopy: | yes/no   if yes, when? ……<br>by who? ………… | |
| Colonic irrigation: | yes/no<br>if yes, when? ………… | |
| Complementary medicine: | yes/no<br>if yes, which area?……<br>since when? ………… | |
| Homeopathic therapy: | yes/no<br>if yes, which globules? ………<br>what strength? ………… | |

| | | |
|---|---|---|
| Schüßler salts: | yes/no<br>if yes, which? .........<br>since when? ............ | |
| Spagyrics: | yes/no<br>if yes, which? ........<br>since when? ......... | |
| Bach flowers therapy: | yes/no<br>if yes, which? ........<br>since when? ............ | |
| Water therapies: | yes/no<br>if yes: silver water<br>magnetite<br>other healing stones | |
| Relaxation exercises: | yes/no<br>if yes: Jacobsen's exercises<br>other | |
| Autogenic training: | yes/no<br>if yes: Prof Dietrich Langen's<br>method   other | |
| Mental/memory exercises: | yes/no<br>if yes, which<br>games/exercises? ............<br>per week: ............ | |
| Dr Clark's zapper: | yes/no<br>if yes,<br>with/without chip programme | |
| M. Frischknecht's<br>TENS device: | yes/no<br>if yes, since when?............ | |
| Dr Clark's liver cleanse: | yes/no<br>if yes, last time: ...... | |

| | | |
|---|---|---|
| Removal of gall stones without surgery: | yes/no<br>if yes, last time: ......... (Dr Clark's method) | |
| Dental reflexology: | yes/no<br>if yes, last time: ......... | |
| Removal of amalgam : | yes/no<br>if yes, when?.................. | |
| Foot reflexology: | yes/no<br>if yes, since when?.... ......... | |
| Singing bowl therapy: | yes/no<br>if yes, since when?............ | |
| Healing stones: | yes/no<br>if yes, which? ............... | |
| Alkaline therapies: | yes/no<br>if yes, which alkaline rinses?......................... | |
| Alkaline baths: | yes/no<br>if yes: baunscheidt therapy<br>alkaline socks    other | |
| $H_2O_2$ (3% hydrogen peroxide): | yes/no<br>if yes, which area?<br>.................. | |
| Wraps: | yes/no<br>if yes: liver wrap<br>herbal wrap    quark wrap | |
| Oil/ointment massages: | yes/no<br>if yes: liver    gall bladder<br>spleen        other | |

| Diet: | alkaline diet: yes/no<br>vegetarian: yes/no<br>vegan: yes/no<br>supplements: yes/no | |
|---|---|---|
| Orthomolecular medicine: | yes/no<br>if yes, which? ............ | |
| Checked house: | yes/no<br>if yes: removal of general disruptions<br>in bedroom  in workroom | |
| Creativity: | yes/no<br>if yes: music    painting<br>craft | |
| Exercise: | yes/no<br>if yes: walking gymnastics<br>golf   muscle training<br>trampolining | |
| Other: | | |

# Work sheet 3
# Initial detoxification programme

Spa therapy at home

Begin with 3–4 weeks of therapy, then take a 3–4 week break, then repeat.

The therapies should be carried out every day without breaks:

Immediately after getting up: one 0.2l glass of pure water, such as healing stone water (e.g. Volvic or Evian with quartz, rose quartz, sodalite and/or similar) made the evening before or mineral water from the brands Leonhardsquelle or Staatlich Fachingen.

Wait 10 minutes

1 glass of water with previously added healing clay, for example Luvos Healing Clay

Wait 10 minutes

1 glass of 'green drink' per day: add 2 tablespoons of *Schoeneberger Saft* – either the horsetail, dandelion, artichoke or nettle version (alternate each day) – to water

Wait 10 minutes

Create a bath:

1½ teaspoons of Luvos Healing Clay and a dash of cider vinegar; alternate daily with a *Sixtus Schlick* bath (or a bath with horsetail: put one handful of horsetail in a saucepan with 2l of water and bring to the boil then simmer for 10 minutes, pass the water through a sieve and add to the bath water). Bathe for 20–30 minutes, then rest for 20–30 to allow post-therapy sweating.

Drink the juice of one freshly squeezed organic pink grapefruit or organic lemon and/or bottled fresh juice such as blackcurrant (check vitamin content) or alternate with other juice (base dosage on information on the label for bottled fresh juices).

Wait 10 minutes

Breakfast

Fresh fruit, freshly cooked sugar-free apple compote, softened dried fruit (must not use sulphur dioxide as a preservative; only use the best quality). Regularly drink glasses of water (as described above) throughout the morning; at least 2l per day in total.

Lunch

A light warm meal with vegetables, etc.
Eat small portions.
In summer water melon can be a good meal occasionally.

In the afternoon

Herbal tea diluted with water and wholemeal bread

In the evening

Herbal tea with water or a clear soup (e.g. onion or similar) and a little wholemeal bread, quark with shoots or similar

During the therapy alcohol, coffee, black tea, meat, processed meats and smoking should be avoided completely.

# Work sheet 4
## What really helps us

You should rate each day. This will allow you to see that the gaps between particularly bad days become longer over time.

Measure pH at least once a day at around 7 a.m. (keep a record); several times a day at specific times in the beginning.


Sun, light and air

Determine the Bovis units (BU) of food and drink using a pendulum. Do not consume anything with under 6500 BU as this weakens the body; consume good, energy-rich food with 9000 BE or 900 nm and above. [You can learn how to use the pendulum through special courses offered by therapists, for example. Our self-help organisation *Selbsthilfeorganisation elementares Wissen e. V.* runs regular pendulum (radionics) courses (see www.elementares-wissen.de).]

Any kind of natural food is always the best choice

Alkaline and acidic food: It is important to pay attention to these two food groups; make sure you know the values of alkaline and acidic foods. The ideal combination is two thirds alkaline and one third of the more acidic foods. For example, combine 'acidic' saltwater fish (acidic because it has a lower pH value) with alkaline vegetables, potatoes, fruit, etc. If you eat a little chocolate or drink a cup of coffee from time to time, this should be balanced out over the course of the day with alkaline water or alkaline teas. You do not need to strictly adhere to the 2:1 ratio for every meal, however; what is important is the overall daily consumption. Over time you will find the right balance.

Water

Spring water from artesian sources is recommended. At artesian sources the

water flows to the surface by itself. This is the case for all healing springs.
Only drink still water such as Volvic, Evian, Chaudfontaine or Courmayeur.
Enrich your water with healing stones and 12 drops of 3% hydrogen
peroxide ($H_2O_2$) per litre. Drinking a glass of water before taking an exam is
supposed to improve grades.
Colloidal water (silver water) can be used as a natural antibiotic when
necessary.

Eat energy-rich food

Organic food and market produce such as carrots, celery, potatoes, radishes,
beetroot, garlic and red onions are essential.
All types of cabbage and, in particular, broccoli contain sulforaphane, which
boosts the immune system. This, in combination with the glucosinolates
found in large quantities in broccoli, savoy cabbage, cauliflower, white
cabbage, radishes and cress, is especially good for the immune system.
These foods are most effective when raw or lightly cooked. Do not cook them
for too long.
Sulforaphane is a compound that is known to be able to kill cancer cells and
prevent toxins and germs in the body causing harm. It has been shown to
protect against breast, cervical, bowel, stomach and prostate cancer.
As it functions as a free radical interceptor, sulforaphane is highly beneficial
for people with weak immune systems due to, for example, fibromyalgia,
cysts and other chronic diseases, as well as severe stress and poor diet.
Potatoes are one of the most beneficial foods, especially blue varieties
(e.g. Vitelotte or Blue Salad Potato). All potato varieties are rich in vitamin
B6 and vitamin C, as well as minerals and trace elements such as
magnesium, iron, potassium and chromium. Enzymes convert energy in
glucose into energy for the body in order to supply the brain and nerves.
The health benefits of potatoes are particularly strong when they are boiled
or steamed.
Fresh nasturtium flowers make an attractive and healthy garnish. The
whole flower should be eaten.
Important: Always chew food thoroughly and break it down into small
pieces. This is good for the stomach and the chewing motion also stimulates

the brain.

### Herbal teas

7 x 7 herbal tea, green oat straw tea, centaurium, dill, nasturtium, buckwheat, yarrow, tarragon, caraway seed, ground ivy, olive leaf.
Willow herb tea is particularly recommended for prostate disease. Drink two cups cold spread out during the day. After three weeks you should notice considerable relief of symptoms.[53]

### Sweetener

Only use raw cane sugar, honey or, better still, stevia as a sweetener. The Stevia rebaudiana plant provides the most natural sweetener in the world and is almost calorie free. This makes stevia particularly suitable for diabetics as it does not affect blood sugar. Dried stevia leaves are available to buy and it is also easy to grow yourself.

### Herbs and spices

Only use organic herbs if possible: marjoram, rosemary, thyme, basil, tarragon, caraway seed, mustard, yeast, garlic, nutmeg, cloves, Ceylon cinnamon, ginger, turmeric and cayenne pepper, as well as fresh peppers and chilies are all recommended.
Salt, which is important for the brain cells, ensures balanced levels of serotonin and melatonin. This helps promote a positive self-image. Nevertheless, you should only use small amounts of salt. When salt is required, I only use energy-rich fleur de sel.
For seasoning I use organic vegetable stock (gluten free, no glutamate, no flavour enhancers, etc.).

### Vegetable juices

Only drink organic juice if possible. Vegetable juices can be diluted with water.
Adding a drop of pumpkin seed oil or virgin olive oil to sauerkraut, carrot, celery, beetroot, potato, radish or vegetable juice is recommended as the body can process the minerals from these vegetables especially well with a

little fat.

Kanne Brottrunk

This product is highly recommended as it promotes health and helps prevent diseases.

Fruit juices

Only drink organic juice if possible or bottled fresh juice, for example blackcurrant, cherry, red grapefruit, orange and sand thorn, blueberry, mangosteen, etc.
Always drink these juices diluted with high quality water.
Check their vitamin and mineral content and compare different manufacturers.
Drink diluted cider vinegar.
Alternating between different fruit and vegetable juices is recommended.
Never drink the same drink for weeks at a time.

Grains

Only use organic grains: millet, barley, spelt, oats, unripe Grünkern spelt, gluten-free buckwheat. They contain large amounts of protein and starch for the nerves and blood vessels. Lupin flour, an alternative to soy flour, contains 16 important amino acids and vitamin E but only a small amount of fat. Chickpea flour is particularly rich in energy. I often use it for baking, mixed with spelt flour or another wholegrain flour. An Italian socca made from chickpea flour with fresh rosemary and good olive oil is delicious and easy to make.

Muesli

Only eat organic muesli. Ideally mix it yourself according to taste, using brown top millet, for example. Brown top millet is the most vitamin-rich grain on Earth. It is gluten free and has large quantities of silicic acid for the skin, hair and nails. It also contains natural fluorine, phosphorus, iron, magnesium, potassium and zinc, as well as the B vitamins B1, B2, B6 and B17. Buckwheat flour is also suitable.

Yellow nutsedge provides magnesium, calcium, protein, vitamin E and unsaturated fats. It is ideal as a snack.
Grape seed flour is rich in proanthocyanidins, acts as an antioxidant and is supposed to be even more effective than grape seed oil. Its antioxidant effect is 50 times stronger than vitamin E and 20 times stronger than vitamin C. Amaranth contains zinc and a third more fibre than wheat. It stores twice as much iron compared to whole grain wheat, as well as high quantities of magnesium, calcium and lysine. Above average amounts of lysine are found in amaranth, which also contains unsaturated fats, linoleic acid and the omega-3 fatty acid alpha-linoleic acid. Black sesame seeds, a common ingredient in Ayurvedic cooking, help bone formation. They are good for combatting osteoporosis and strengthen the liver and kidneys.
Oats are the best and cheapest source of vitamins. Large, natural oats should be eaten instead of bread, if not all then some of the time.
Other possible ingredients include linseed, spelt bran, blonde psyllium, Edelhefe oats, grain mixes, nuts, seeds, various fruits, pollen, honey, and many more.

Meat

Little or none; a maximum of 300g of meat products per week. If you do eat meat, choose free range products such as poultry (e.g. chicken), lamb or rabbit, which should of course be organic. Ensure that the animals were reared naturally without added hormones, genetically modified feed, antibiotics or other pharmaceutical products.

Saltwater fish

Suitable if the fish is caught from the sea. You should be wary of heavy metal contamination of tuna and swordfish; for this reason it should only be eaten occasionally and in small quantities. This also applies to some saltwater fish from certain regions. Unfortunately, consumers usually only hear about contamination through local media, such as if a nearby river or lake has been contaminated by pollutants or poisonous waste such as large quantities of pesticides.
Oysters are a good source of zinc but are not alkaline; nevertheless, they are beneficial because of their minerals, like saltwater fish. The low pH value

should be balanced out with other alkaline foods.
I avoid farmed fish as it is often treated with artificial hormones and
antibiotics and fed genetically modified food.

Cheese

Only eat organic, unpasteurised varieties if possible – without any additives
such as colourings, flavourings, preservatives and other E numbers. I avoid
cheeses that have been pasteurised or treated with heat as the vitamins and
minerals are no longer able to take their full effect after heating.
Unfortunately, there are no longer many unpasteurised cheeses available,
but those that do exist are particularly aromatic. The best kinds, if you like
the taste, are unpasteurised sheep or goat cheese. Unpasteurised cheese
is clearly labelled as such.

Fruit and berries

Only eat organic varieties if possible. There is a huge variety to choose from:
blueberries, rose hip, elderberries, sand thorn, acerola cherries, apples,
papaya, pineapples, mangos, goji berries, passion fruit, mangosteen,
raspberries, blackcurrants, cranberries, pomegranates, schisandra berries,
apricots, aronia berries and many more are all healthy and tasty. Oranges – if
possible blood oranges from Sicily because the lava-enriched soil contains
particularly large amounts of minerals – and pink grapefruits are especially
good. Eat the seeds as well, making sure you chew them thoroughly. They are
supposed to help prevent cancer, as are raspberries.
Dried fruits (as long as they do not use sulphur dioxide as a preservative)
such as plums, dates, figs, raisins or apricots are also recommended.
Raspberries and blackberries contain large amounts of iron, magnesium,
calcium and phosphorus. They are particularly good at regulating the
metabolism, and support nerve and brain function and liver purification.

Vegetables and grains

Only eat organic varieties if possible. There are many to choose from:
parsley, sauerkraut, red cabbage, wild garlic, peppers, white and black
radishes, beetroot, potatoes, horseradish, garlic, onions, red radishes,
turnips,

artichokes, celery, all types of cabbage, brown rice (especially varieties of rice from the Camargue or Japan), nori seaweed.

Seeds and nuts

Only eat organic varieties if possible. All kinds are recommended, provided you are not allergic to any of them: sunflower seeds, nettle seeds, milk thistle seeds, pumpkin seeds, parsley seeds, cardamom. They are particularly important for increasing brain activity.
Walnuts, almonds, cashews, peanuts (with the skin), coconuts, hazelnuts and chestnuts are also recommended. Warning: You should be especially careful to ensure that there is no mould on nuts.

Oils

Only use the best organic oils: virgin olive oil, wheat germ oil, evening primrose oil, grapeseed oil, pumpkinseed oil, etc.

Oxygen $H_2O_2$

Vitamins

Make sure vitamins are natural. The following cover the daily requirements:
All the B vitamins are important, especially B1, B2, B3, B6 and B12.
B3 is found in oats, wheat germ and eggs, for example. 25–100 mg of B6 activates brain cell activity, particularly in combination with zinc. 5–10 µg of B12 supports the brain and nerves. It is found in liver, oysters, spirulina, organic salmon, herring and sauerkraut, for example. It can also be taken as a vitamin B complex supplement.
Your daily vitamin C intake should initially be up to 1 000 mg (but do not consume more than 500mg at once, otherwise it will be removed unused). Warning: Do not consume ascorbic acid (synthetic vitamin C); only consume vitamin C in its biological form.
Vitamin E: Daily intake should be up to 500 mg. Look out for the name tocopherol.
Vitamin D: 3–10 µg plus lecithin

Minerals

Only use the best quality minerals (determine with a pendulum if necessary).
Selenium: Determine individual values through kinesiological testing.
50–100 µg per day is normal. Warning: Too much selenium is toxic.
Magnesium: 100–250 mg
Ginkgo: good for memory, stops symptoms of dementia
Folic acid: 0.3–1 mg; found in eggs, spinach, etc.
Phosphorus: found in celery, egg yolk, cheese, salmon, nuts, wheat germ, pulses
Chromium: 30–150 µg; found in garlic, whole wheat, yeast, grain oils
Iodine: 150–300 µg; found in seafood, eggs, papaya, mango, pineapple
Manganese: 2–6 mg; found in nuts, olives, blueberries, sunflower seeds, avocado, spinach
Zinc: 10–20 mg; found in oysters, liver, spirulina, lentils, nuts, meat
Chlorella: algae that remove heavy metals
Spirulina: algae that contains many vitamins and removed toxins
AFA klamath: This algae should be wild; it contains 22 amino acids, vitamins B1, B2, B3, B5, B6, and B12, folic acid, vitamin C and vitamin E. It has a direct effect on the brain, helping against poor concentration and memory problems.
Chlorophyll: improves brain function; found in barley grass juice, barley juice tablets, spelt grass tablets, all algae, especially chlorella
Gamma-linolenic acid: for better blood fat levels
Clinoptilolite: incredibly finely ground volcanic rock that removes toxins and heavy metals
Coenzyme Q10: 200–400 mg
Wheat germ oil: high vitamin E content
Primrose oil: very good for the skin
Grape seed extract: proanthocyanidins are a good antioxidant and promote blood flow to the brain.
Siberian ginseng: reduces listlessness
Hawthorn: promotes blood flow throughout the body
Copper and zinc: particularly important minerals for all brain diseases

Omega 3 fatty acids
Niacin (vitamin B3): a good addition for improving blood flow

# Tips for an active and healthy life

Energy transfer with elementary meditation: transfer lacking energy; i.e. healing through the power of thoughts

Meditation, prayer

Autogenic training

Breathing: learn to breathe deeply and consciously; abdominal breathing and/or deep breaths in and out with arms wide

Vigorous chewing; each chewing motion stimulates the brain; jaw muscle training

Dr Kawashima's brain exercises

Atlas correction

Orthopaedic shoes (e.g. MBT shoes)

Magnetic field therapy

Dark field microscopy accompanied by homeopathic medication

Rechtsregulat: in the morning and evening, hold in your mouth for a long time

Remove all forms of toxification such as heavy metals, overacidification, viruses, fungi leeches, worms, etc. (obtain diagnosis of the blood terrain using dark field microscopy)

Oxygen therapy, autohaemotherapy

Garlic cure: twice a year

Vitamins, minerals, orthomolecular medicine

Aslan therapy

Alkaline baths (full, foot or arm) using Dr Jentschura's method (progress slowly); every day take a warm shower followed by a cold shower and massage the entire body with a brush working towards the excretory organs, use a baunscheidt roller
Alkaline shirt, stockings, hat, neck wraps, liver wraps, etc.; alkaline rinsing of the sinuses, inhaling, alkaline diet, alkaline enemas: once every 14 days, after 3 months only once a month

Ayurvedic detoxification, Ayurvedic lifestyle

Heavy metal detoxification of the blood (have amalgam and dead teeth removed)

Dental reflexology

Foot reflexology

Complementary medicine: Dr Clark's zapper[54]; Martin Frischknecht's TENS device and Powertube[55]; liver purification and gall stone removal: once or twice a year

Homeopathy (Dr Jentschura's methods)[56]: Kalium chloratum D6, Silicea D12, Calcium phosphoricum D6 and others

Schüßler salts (Kellenberger's method)[57]: no. 2 Calcium phosphoricum, no. 4 Kalium, no. 11 Silicea D12; a pendulum can be used to determine others

Bach flower remedies: no. 13 Gorse, no. 21 Mustard, no. 23 Olive, no. 30 Sweet Chestnut, no. 27 Rock Water[58]

Acupuncture/acupressure: chakra, meridians, chi
Relax and energise the central nervous system using Mr Thai's method with special sticks or meditation, for example
Meridian points: left and/or bottom right of the back of the head, transformer, also called Medulla oblongata (subchakra), the lower edge of the skull and top of the cervical spine, hands, back, feet and the point of the central nervous system in the middle of the head
Acupressure: in case of tremor, for example, on the back of the head/edge of the skull (see meridian points and ear acupuncture)

Singing bowl meditation: ideally with old bowls made of alloys consisting of 12 different metals

Healing stones: jasper, topaz, emerald, citrine, mookaite, chalcedony

Breuss' rubs and wraps[59] and anthroposophic medicine

Physiotherapy, speech therapy, occupational therapy, music therapy at least once a week

Daily exercises at home

Feldenkrais therapy: one additional session per week

Liver wraps, kidney wraps

Liver purification: once a year

Colon hydrotherapy, colon cleansing

Coordination exercises

Dorn-Breuss spinal therapy

Yoga

Creative hobbies such as painting and/or playing an instrument, dancing, listening to music

Exercise such as trampolining, power plate, golf

Walking, walking taking large steps

Laughter: try laughter yoga

Strength training such as Kieser training: gently and in moderation so that acids do not build up in the muscles

Very important: the right bed

Remove disruptions in the home, bedroom and living space (with the help of a geophysicist if necessary)

Pillow filled with spelt or millet

Self-discipline

Constantly strengthen the will

Movement, movement, movement ...

In addition:
Apply for a disability badge

To be avoided:
Long periods watching television

Long periods working on a computer

Driving for long periods of time

Using the telephone (land-line or mobile) – turn Wi-Fi off when not in use

Poor diet with chemical additives

Toxins in wood protector, pesticides and other toxic materials

Alcohol

Tobacco

Negative thoughts

Conflict

Hate

Envy

Jealousy

Stress


If you have any questions, further information or comments, please contact:
Selbsthilfeorganisation elementares Wissen e. V.

www.elementares-wissen.de
info@elementares-wissen.de

Thank you for your help!

# Afterword

I have tried therapies 1 to 32 in part II myself. I have organised them in order of importance based on my current perspective. It is very likely that not all therapies will be necessary in each individual case, but as we cannot know in advance what is right for each individual, it makes sense to test them. For this reason, harmful side effects are not generally to be expected.

For me the most important step in the healing process was the meditation therapy which led me to other treatments (see part I, 2007).
My first step towards physical healing was Atlas correction which, when done correctly, is only required once. My first successful treatments for cleansing my organs were the detoxification course (see work sheet 4) and later the Breuss treatment. Then came deacidification – a big and very important topic. By this point I had switched completely to an alkaline diet and alkaline lifestyle.
It was over two years before I discovered heavy metal detoxification and came to the realisation that heavy metals make the brain ill.

The results of the examinations using dark field microscopy and the comprehensive professional advice from my alternative practitioner finally led me to a breakthrough in 2009. This was the first time that my Parkinson's factor was decreased noticeably.
In my case, the heavy metal deposits, typical of Parkinson's disease, were evidence of many years of excessive exposure. Despite methods to cleanse my body of heavy metals in 2004 and 2005 my efforts were unsuccessful.

Why? The mutated intestinal flora had caused the metals to become
embedded in my body and in my brain. I then took a very strict course of
homeopathic medication.
A crucial advantage for me was the changes that I had already made to my
lifestyle, including switching to an alkaline lifestyle. This meant that much of
the excessive acidification in my body had already been corrected.
Today, in 2012, you can no longer notice or see signs of Parkinson's disease
in me. Nevertheless, I know that a little of it is still there. When I talk for a
longer period of time saliva still accumulates in my mouth; my swallowing
reflex is still a little delayed. The neural pathways for swallowing have
suffered.
My sense of smell is also still not back to how it used to be. Nevertheless, it
has returned to a sufficient extent that I am able to detect the warning
signal of a bad smell coming from something that is dangerous to me. But if
this is the only handicap, I can call myself healthy today. My 'old' diseases
such as the chronic polyarthritis, fibromyalgia, arthrosis in my knees,
headaches and the initial signs of an ulcer, some of which I had been
fighting with medication since my childhood, have disappeared since I
changed over to a lifestyle that is more of less free of toxins, changed my
diet and developed my new sense of spirituality.

For this reason I ask you: trust yourself and your own spiritual guidance! Be
open and open yourself to methods of healing that might seem unusual to
you right now. Find an experienced alternative practitioner or naturopath
who has experience with your disease. And remain critical. Look for people
who want to heal you. It will not cost a fortune. If you are asked to pay in
advance this should make you suspicious.
You will be able to feel it yourself. Only absolute trust will allow you to
make progress.

Some of the topics in this book do not seem relevant to Parkinson's disease
at first glance. However, when looking at them for a second time it becomes
clear that health and disease should be considered as a whole from a physical,
mental and spiritual perspective. When seeing things from this point of view,
many factors that remained unconsidered before gain increased importance.

The unhealthy environments we have created for ourselves and the toxins that we expose ourselves to through poor diet and bad habits, for example, act like poison in our bodies – whether we want them to or not.
We can think of health as a complex mosaic or puzzle. Each mosaic tile or puzzle piece has its function. If one piece is missing, the full picture is not complete. Diseases fill the gaps, attack the surrounding pieces, continuing until we are too weak to do anything to prevent it.

So what about the observations I made at the beginning of this book, the parallels that I drew? My observations are even more horrifying than I could have imaged.
According to information from the USA, the number of incidences of Parkinson's disease is set to rise dramatically. I believe that this increase is related to the ever increasing presence of heavy metals, such as mercury, lead and aluminium, chemical preparations, and industrial food that is lacking in minerals, along with rising pollution.

Until now, Parkinson's disease has mainly affected people between 50 and 60 years of age, but according to current reports in the media it is now affecting more and more people in their 40s, and the age limit is set to decrease even further. This corresponds to my experience.

This essentially confirms the conclusion that I presented at the beginning of this book: civilisation today is a cause of Parkinson's and many other diseases. Food that contains unnecessary chemical additives, synthetic medications, tremendous amounts of radiation, constant light, permanent noise, hyper activity and many other things are all causes of the slow weakening of our health and 'feed' many diseases.

We are called to reflect, to 'reduce', to become happy, content and healthy again. But we must take responsibility for this.

I am sure that God led me to all of these experiences and findings. And now I know why.

I am thankful for that.

# My self-help organisation: *Selbsthilfeorganisation elementares Wissen e. V.*

In thanks for my spiritual and physical healing after many years with Parkinson's disease, I fulfilled my promise of establishing an independent charitable self-help organisation. The purpose and goal of this organisation is to allow all sick people, without exception, to receive and truly experience love and compassion. The organisation's name is simply *elementares Wissen* – elementary knowledge.

### The organisation's goals

The organisation's guiding principle comes from Hippocrates of Cos: Let food be your medicine, and medicine be your food!
This means spreading elementary knowledge about a healthy diet and the possibilities of healing offered by modern natural medicine, and spreading basic knowledge about a healthy lifestyle and how to maintain health based on ancient examples and modern findings.

The independent charitable organisation supports individuals so that those who are ill or look after those who are ill may be able to benefit from the most elementary things in life. It helps educate independent self-help groups, as independent self-help organisations and groups are in the best position to pass the best, unbiased information on to people.

The knowledge of all medical experts specialised in research and teaching and the therapeutic knowledge of all doctors, all naturopathists and all alternative practitioners, but also the experiences of laypeople can be very helpful for this purpose. In our self-help organisation, everyone involved has the same right to share their thoughts and information.

The organisation supports the establishment of networks. These
networks allow the best possible, unbiased information to be
distributed to those affected.

The programme

Information services and provision of useful addresses
Publicity
Seminars on an alkaline lifestyle, heavy metal toxification
and many more topics; courses on recognising food
(learning to distinguish what is better!) and much more;
individual sessions
The independent charitable organisation *Selbsthilfeorganisation
elementares Wissen e. V.* aims to spread the word about natural
medicine in teaching and research.
What exactly do we do?
One of our tasks will be to develop a prize that will be awarded to
individuals, universities, specialist schools, institutions or research
groups that have the skills and the courage to publish new findings,
and are not afraid to make complementary medicine available to
patients as a holistic, scientific form of medicine.
The organisation offers help and support. In doing so, it considers the
possibilities of natural medicine and other forms of complementary,
holistic medicine in as much detail as the possibilities of conventional
medicine.
The organisation is open to everyone, regardless of religion, culture,
skin colour or nationality. It is entirely non-profit. It aims to be
selfless and does not have any financial interests.


## Helping makes people happy!

The independent and charitable organisation *Selbsthilfeorganisation
elementares Wissen e. V.* does not aim to be an alternative to
chemical treatment. Instead, it aims for dual, holistic, integrated
therapy. If we embrace life, have a clear mind and use the power of

our thoughts, we can achieve anything.

If you share my belief, I invite you to support my self-help organisation *Selbsthilfeorganisation elementares Wissen e. V.*, either as an active member or financial supporter. Please write to us and tell us how you would like to be involved. Alternatively, if you need help, please explain your worries or your illnesses. You are also very welcome to contact us if you would like to share your opinions and experiences with the organisation, for example in the form of a seminar or presentation.

If you would like to support our organisation, you can find more information on our website, www.elementares-wissen.de.

*Selbsthilfeorganisation elementares Wissen e. V.* was officially registered in Germany as a non-profit organisation on 22 June 2011 (Amtsgericht Arnsberg VR no. 1295; Finanzamt Brilon).

If you have any questions or suggestions regarding the organisation, please write to info@elementares-wissen.de.

You data will be treated confidentially and not used for any other purposes.

# I would like to say thank you!

My thanks goes to all the doctors who helped me to identify my Parkinson's disease. My thanks goes to all the doctors who supported me and encouraged me during my search for possibilities of finding help without chemical and pharmacological preparations.

My thanks goes to all the alternative practitioners, therapists and specialists in natural medicine who have helped me to achieve true health.

My thanks goes to all the teachers of meditation and wisdom who were able to promote a natural knowledge of the powers and possibilities of the universe in me to allow me to use this knowledge for myself and for other people in a practical way.

My thanks goes to all the authors, publishers and broadcasters who generously allowed me to quote their work which enriches this book.

My thanks goes to all my friends and family who have accompanied and supported me with my projects, which may have been strange at times, who simply always hoped along with me that one day everything would turn into something good.

# Appendix

# Information and addresses

Selbsthilfeorganisation elementares Wissen e. V. Am Kreuzberg 9
59955 Winterberg
Germany
www.elementares-wissen.de

DKD – Deutsche Klinik für Diagnostik 65191
Wiesbaden
Germany
www.dkd-wiesbaden.de

Anthrosana – Verein für anthroposophisch erweitertes Heilwissen
4144 Arlesheim
Switzerland
www.anthrosana.ch

S.E.M. – Seminare für elementare Meditation Am Kreuzberg 9
59955 Winterberg
Germany
www.elementare-meditation.de

Thai N. B.-Zentrum 6015
Reussbühl

Switzerland
www.tnbluzern.ch

Addresses of manufacturers and distributors

For the manufacturer addresses, please contact my independent self-help organisation, *Selbsthilfeorganisation elementares Wissen e. V.* (www.elementares-wissen.de)


Useful websites

Atlas correction: www.atlasprofilax.ch
Dr Markus Sommer: www.gesundheitaktiv-heilkunst.de
IG Dunkelfelddiagnostik: www.ig-df.de
Dentalreflex: www.dentalreflex.ch
Genetic research – Umweltinstitut München: www.umweltinstitut.org
Greenpeace – fishing: www.greenpeace.de/themen/meere/fischerei
Stiftung nano-control, Hamburg: www.nano-control.de
Conscious eating – nutritional information: www.foodwatch.de
Product tests: www.oekotest.de
Consumer information: www.lebensmittelklarheit.de
Healing stones and minerals: www.mineralientage.de
Chelation therapy: www.chelat.biz
PSP: www.psp-gesellschaft.de
Dark field microscopy: www.naturheilpraxis-scheller.de
Feldenkrais therapy: www.feldenkraisliga.de
Greenpeace – genetic engineering: www.greenpeace.de/themen/gentechnik
Bundesverband Patienten für Homöopathie e. V.: www.bph-online.de
Natur und Medizin e. V.: www.naturundmedizin.de
Deutsche Homöopathische Union: www.DHU.de
YOGA-Vidya: www.yoga-vidya.de
Light-based technologies: www.biophotonik.org
Deutscher Verband für Physiotherapie: www.zvk.org
www.spiegel.de/wissenschaft/mensch
PM magazine: www.pm-magazin.de
Diagnosis and treatment: www.netdoktor.de
Health information: www.vitagate24.ch

Traditional Chinese medicine: www.tcm-schweiz.ch
Deutsche Akademie für Akupunktur: www.akupunktur.de
Institut für CranioSacral Healing: www.craniosacral-healing.de
Patient information centre: www.parkinsonweb.com
Hospital search: www.weisse-liste.de
Interessengemeinschaft Gesundheit: www.igg.ch
Implant acupuncture: www.inauris.com/parkinson
Patient help: www.washabich.de
Vegetarierbund Deutschland: www.vebu.de
N.I.E.-Netzwerk Impfentscheid: www.impfentscheid.ch

# Footnotes and comments

## Part I

1 Blüchel, Kurt G., *Heilen verboten – töten erlaubt*, p. 388 2
Breuss, Rudolf, *Die Breuss Krebskur*, pp. 37–52 [English
translation published under the title *The Breuss Cancer Cure*]
3 Clark, Dr., H. R. *Heilverfahren aller Krebsarten*
[English original published under the title *The Cure
for all Cancers*]
4 ibid., p. 93
5 ibid., pp. 28–37
6 Emoto, Masuro, *Wasserkristalle*, pp. 16–22 [English translations Emoto's works are also
available]
7 Elmadfa, Prof. Dr., Ibrahim, *E-Nummern*, pp. 20–85
8 Knophius Heike, *Säure-Basen-Balance*, pp. 40–65
9 Beck, Dr. Robert C., *Kolloidales Silber*
10 Hürlimann, Gertrud I., *Rute und Pendel*, pp. 197–200
11 Further information: *sho.elementares-wissen@t-online.de*
12 Welt der Wunder, *Zeitbombe Essen*, November 2010, p. 66
13 Fliege, *Parkinson - Können Nadeln heilen*, December 2007, p. 64
14 Jentschura, Dr. h. c., Peter and Lohkämper, Josef, *Zivilisatoselos;
Gesundheit durch Entschlackung*
15 Welt der Wunder, *Wie wirken die geheimen Kräfte des Magnetismus*,
August 2008, p. 22
16 Welt der Wunder, *Heilen Magnete Krankheiten*, January 2010, p. 57
17 Sharamon Shalila, Baginski, Bodo J., *Die Schisandrabeere*, p. 11, 17 – 1 8 ,
24, 26, 30, 40, 44 – 4 5
18 Information on over 50 Yoga Vidya centres in Germany: www.yoga-
vidya.de.
19 Kühni, W., von Holst, W., *Taschenlexikon der Heilsteine* 20
Fliege, *Parkinson*, April 2008
21 Welt der Wunder, *Wie Musik das Gehirn heilt*, March 2008, pp. 14–23
22 ZDF, 38°, section on Parkinson's disease, June 2008

23 Welt der Wunder, *Magnete contra Alzheimer?*, August 2008, p. 29 24 ARD, Fakt, *Wirkstoffe in Medikamenten*, September 2008

25 ARD, Plusminus, *Seniorenessen*, 3 November 2009

26 Welt der Wunder, *Die Krebskiller aus dem Nano-Universum*, August 2008

27 Welt der Wunder, *Wie gefährlich sind Nano-Teilchen in unserem Essen?*, Feb. 2010, p.87

28 Hürlimann, Gertrud, *Rute und Pendel* 29 Virapen, John, *Nebenwirkung Tod* [English original published under the title *Side Effects: Death*]

30 ibid. p. 254

31 Grün, Sigrid and Neidhardt, Jan, *Aronia*

32 Interview with Karl Gamper, Gala-Spirit, 01/2009

33 Spalding, Baird T., *Leben und Lehren der Meister im fernen Osten, Band 4/5*, p. 294

34 www.ZeitenSchrift.com, 55/07

35 Karstädt, Uwe, *Entgiften statt vergiften*

36 Treben, Maria, *Gesundheit aus der Apotheke Gottes* [English translation published under the title *Health through God's Pharmacy*]

37 Upledger, Dr., John E., *Auf den inneren Arzt hören* [English original published under the title *Your inner physician and you*]

38 Treben, Maria, *Gesundheit aus der Apotheke Gottes*, p. 44, 61, 87 [English translation published under the title *Health through God's Pharmacy*]

39 www.spiegel.de

40 Further information www.ig-df.de

41 Fliege

42 Scheller, Ekkehard and Sabine, *Candidalismus?!*, chap. Symbionten pp. 20–23

43 ibid., chap.11, Spiritueller Ausblick, p. 195

44 ibid., p. 12, pp. 45–55, 56–60

45 Blank, Dr. med., K.-H., Scheller, E., HP, Seidler, J.A., Ganswindt, T., Köhler, Dr. med., A., *»Damit müssen Sie jetzt leben!« NEIN Danke!*, p. 9 – 1 0

46 ibid., pp. 22–32

47 Virapen, John, *Nebenwirkung Tod* [English original published under the title *Side Effects: Death*]

48 Clark, Dr., H. R., *Heilverfahren aller Krebsarten* [English original published under the title *The Cure for all Cancers*]

49 Frischknecht, Martin, *Gesundheit als Chance*, pp. 13–74

50 ibid., p. 80 – 8 1
51 Yoda, Prof. Dr., Peter, *Ein medizinischer Insider packt aus* 52
ibid., p. 147
53 Pschyrembel, *Klinisches Wörterbuch,* p. 1350
54 Shioya, Dr., Nobuo, *Der Jungbrunnen des Dr. Shioya*
55 Herbst, Erika, *Die Lösung des Krebsproblems, Die Heilkunst von Morgen,*
p. 1133
56 ibid., p. 1136
57 ibid., p. 1136
58 Apotheken Umschau, *Besser leben mit Parkinson,* December 2009,
pp.20–24
59 Welt der Wunder, *Die tödliche Macht der Gedanken,* 12/2009, pp. 60–65
60 ibid.
61 ibid.
62 ibid.
63 ibid.
64 ibid.
65 Bösch, Dr. med., PD, Jacob, *Versöhnen und Heilen*
66 reform rundschau 16/2009, Dr. med. Freiherr Jürgen von Rosen, *Was für
ein Schwindel,* p. 12; for further information contact prof.molitor@t-online.de
67 Frischknecht, Martin, *Gesundheit als Chance,* p. 228 68
ibid., p. 230
69 ibid., p. 230
70 Further information: www.alpenparlament.ch, www.vitamins-for-all.org,
www.igg.ch
71 Sharamom, Shalaila, Baginski, Bodo J., *Goji,* p. 11, 15, 48, 94 72
ibid. p. 99
73 ibid. p. 105
74 Jentschura, Dr. h. c., Peter und Lohkämper, Josef, *Zivilisatoselos*
75 Kunhardt von, Gert, *Kleiner aufwand grosse wirkung* 76
ibid. p. 20
77 Further information: sho.elementares-wissen@t-online.de
78 Kuby, Clemens, *Heilung das Wunder in uns,* inside back cover
79 Kuby, Clemens, *Unterwegs in die nächste Dimension,* p. 140

## Part II

1 Jentschura, Dr. h. c., Peter und Lohkämper, Josef, *Gesundheit durch Entschlackung,* chap. Die körperchemische Grundregulation, pp. 28–48

2 Jentschura, Dr. h. c. und Peter, Lohkämper, Josef, *Zivilisatoselos,* chap. Was ist Zivilisatose?, p. 29

3 Jentschura, Dr. h. c., Peter und Lohkämper, Josef, *Zivilisatoselos,* chap., Iß, trink, tue Nützliches!, pp. 132–147

4 Breuss, Rudolf, *Die Breuss Krebskur,* chap. Warum wieder gekochte Speisen wertlos, ja sogar schädlich sein können, p. 99 et. seq. [English translation published under the title *The Breuss Cancer Cure*]

5 Elmadfa, Prof. Dr., Ibrahim, Muskat, Prof. Dr., E., Fritzsche, Dipl. oec. troph., *E-Nummern,* chap. E-Nummern-Liste, pp. 12–72

6 Drogistenstern, Ausg. 7–8/2009, source: wikipedia.org

7 Kellenberger, Richard und Kopsche, Friedrich, *Mineralstoffe nach Dr. Schüssler,* Wie finde ich den richtigen Mineralstoff, p. 227

8 Jentschura, Dr. h. c., Peter und Lohkämper, Josef, *Zivilisatoselos,* chapter Parkinson, p. 349

9 Clark, Dr., H. R., *Heilverfahren aller Krebsarten,* pp. 37-40 [English original published under the title *The Cure for all Cancers*]

10 Frischknecht, Martin, *Gesundheit als Chance,* p. 138–139

11 Breuss, Rudolf, *Die Breuss Krebskur,* p. 38 [English translation published under the title *The Breuss Cancer Cure*]

12 Scheller, Ekkehard und Sabine, *Candidalismus?!,* chap. Schwermetalle, p. 74, p.176

13 Further information: www.heilzentrum-scheller.de, www.ig-df.de

14 Jentschura, Dr. h. c., Peter und Lohkämper, Josef, *Gesundheit durch Entschlackung,* chap. Die zielgerichtete Entschlackung, p. 205

15 Scheller, Ekkehard und Sabine, *Candidalismus?!,* chapter 12: Die Darmflora bestimmt unser inneres Milieu, p. 44

16 Further information: Naturheilpraxis Scheller und Kollegen, Labor für Pleomorphie, Winkl 8, 83115 Neubeuern, Germany

17 Breuss, Rudolf, *Die Breuss Krebskur* [English translation published under the title *The Breuss Cancer Cure*]

18 Karstädt, Uwe, *Entgiften statt vergiften,* chap. Strahlen – die vertuschte Gefahr,

p. 44

19 Further information: Interessengemeinschaft Gesundheit IGG, www.igg.ch

20 Apotheken Umschau , *Chlorfrei Planschen,* 05/2010, p. 46 21 ARD-Sendung Plusminus, 3 February 2009

22 Welt der Wunder, *Autopsie eines Krebserregers,* August 2010, pp. 92–97

23 Further information: Umweltinstitut München e. V., Verein zur Erforschung und Verminderung der Umweltbelastung, Landwehrstr. 64 a, 80336 München, Germany. www.umweltinstitut.org.

24 Further information: foodwatch, Brunnenstr. 181, 10119 Berlin. www.foodwatch.de

25 *Das Ziel muss die Umwandlung aller Gesunden in Kranke sein.* Deutsches Ärzteblatt, 20 September 2002, article: *Der Wettbewerb zwingt zur Erschließung neuer Märkte;* cited from the book by Blüchel, Kurt G., *Heilen verboten – töten erlaubt,* chap. Die organisierte Kriminalität im Gesundheitswesen, p. 299

26 Kühni, Werner, Holst von, Walter, *Taschenlexikon der Heilsteine,* p. 130 27 The ARD television programme *W wie Wissen* presented a report entitled *Hokuspokus mit Heilsteinen* (hocus pocus with healing stones). A professor of mineralogy from the University of Tübingen said in the report that he had never felt the supposed vibration of the stones. Quote (translated from the original German): 'I believe that it is an easy way to get people to part with their money.' The fact that he holds a professorship in mineralogy does not prove that this statement is correct. Are the things that one does *not* know hocus pocus? ARD programme *W wie Wissen, Hokuspokus mit Heilsteinen,* 13 December 2009

28 Feldenkrais, Moshé, *Abenteuer im Dschungel des Gehirns* 29 www.yoga-vidya.de

30 Breuss, Rudolf, *Die Breuss Krebskur,* chap. Schmerzloses, Wirbelsäuleneinrichten nach Rudolf Breuss, pp. 103–105 [English translation published under the title *The Breuss Cancer Cure*]

31 Raslan, Gamal, *Der sanfte Weg zur Mitte: Die Dorn-Methode*

32 Fleig, Harald, *Heilen über die Wirbelsäule,* www.breuss-dorn-therapie.de

33 Bärenklau, Drs. med. dent., Beatrix und Uwe, presentation held in 2009 at the first Appenzeller Gesundheitskongress, Schwellbrunn, Switzerland. www.dentalreflex.de

34 Welt der Wunder, *Die geheimen Bahnen der Körperenergien Meridiane,* January 2010 issue, pp. 54–56

35 Friedrich Schiller University Jena, Institute of Physical Chemistry,

Forschungsschwerpunkt Biophotonik, Prof. Dr. Jürgen Popp, Helmholtzweg 4, 07743 Jena, www.biophotonik.org

36 Further information: Behandlungs-Zentrum Energie-Fokussierung Luzern, Thai, Ngoc-Buu, Fluhmühlerain 2, 6015 Reussbühl Lu, Switzerland. www. tnbluzern.ch

37 Upledger, Dr., John E., *Auf den inneren Arzt hören* [English original published under the title *Your inner physician and you*]

38 Further information: www.cranioverband.org, www.aslan.info/aktuell/physiotherapie.html, www.thalamus.de

39 Bach, Dr., Edward, *Heile Dich selbst mit den Bachblüten*

40 Jentschura, Dr. h. c., Peter and Lohkämper, Josef, *Zivilisatoselos,* chapter Parkinson, Naturheilkunde, p. 349

41 Karstädt, Uwe, *Entgiften statt vergiften,* p. 23, pp. 50–57

42 ibid., p. 11, 37

43 ibid., p. 139

44 Further information: www.uwekarstaedt.de

45 ibid., p. 47

46 ibid., pp. 50–57

47 Scheller, Ekkehard und Sabine, *Candidalismus?!,* chapter Schwermetalle (Teil 1), p. 79–80

48 S.E.M. Seminare für elementare Meditation, Am Kreuzberg 9, 59955 Winterberg, Germany, www.elementare-meditation.de

49 Selbsthilfeorganisation elementares Wissen e.V., Am Kreuzberg 9, 59955 Winterberg, Germany, www.elementares-wissen.de

50 Fintelmann, Prof. Dr. med., Volker, *Parkinson-Krankheit,* issue 207, anthrosana

51 Verein für anthroposophisch erweitertes Heilwesen e.V., Johannes-Kepler-Str. 56, 75378 Bad Liebenzell, Germany. www.heilwesen.de

52 Scheller, Ekkehard und Sabine, *Candidalismus?!*

53 Welt der Wunder, *Mikronährstoffe – wie gefährlich machen sie mein Es-sen?,* January 2010 issue, p. 67

54 Jentschura, Dr. h. c., Peter und Lohkämper, Josef, *Zivilisatoselos,* chapter Die Kuhmilch, p. 118

55 Clark, Dr., H. R., *Heilverfahren aller Krebsarten,* chapter Werden Sie wieder gesund, p. 89 [English original published under the title *The Cure for all Cancers*]

56 Welt der Wunder, *Was das Essen mit uns macht. Der große Lebensmit-teltest,* issue 2/2008, pp. 54–62

57 ZDF-Frontal 21, *Politiker verhindern Schulobst*, 26.01.2010

58 Welt der Wunder, *Wie gefährlich sind Nano-Teilchen in unserem Essen?*, issue 2/2010, pp. 86–91

59 ibid., pp. 86–91

60 ibid.

61 Karstädt, Uwe, *Entgiften statt vergiften*, p. 140, 223

62 ibid., p. 152

63 See part III, work sheets and summary

64 Jentschura, Dr. h. c., Peter und Lohkämper, Josef, *Zivilisatoselos*, chapter Die Impfungen, p. 125

65 Karstädt, Uwe, *Entgiften statt vergiften*, Vorwort, p. 11

66 Aktories, Forstermann, *Lehrbuch der Pharmakologie und Toxikologie*, Hofmann/Starke, 2005, p. 845, in *Feuerwerk Leben*, 1/2010

67 Comprehensive information about influenza vaccinations and other vaccinations: AEGIS Schweiz, Daniel Trappitsch, www.impfforum.ch

68 Further information: www.vaccsecure.com, www.neue-medizin.com/ impfpok.htm

69 Jentschura, Dr. h. c., Peter, Lohkämper, Josef, *Zivilisatoselos*, chap. Die Impfungen, p. 128f., Robert-Koch-Institut, Paul-Ehrlich-Institut

70 Karstädt, Uwe, *Entgiften statt vergiften*, Vorwort, p. 11 and chap. Vergiftet und Gegessen, p. 30

71 ibid., Appendix D, p. 268

72 Clark, Dr., H. R., *Heilverfahren aller Krebsarten*, p. 104, 191, 196, 245, 269, 305, 317, 348, 358, 359, 360, 377, 491, 492, 534, 535 [English original published under the title *The Cure for all Cancers*]

73 Jentschura, Dr. h. c., Peter, Lohkämper, Josef, *Zivilisatoselos*, chapter Meide Schädliches, p. 94f., chap. Base statt Deo, p. 163, 172

74 ibid., p. 98

75 Frischknecht, Martin, *Gesundheit als Chance*, chap. Giftstoffe, p. 204

76 Jentschura, Dr. h. c., Peter, Lohkämper, Josef, *Zivilisatoselos*, chap. Meide Schädliches, p. 98

77 Bärenklau, Drs. med. dent., Uwe und Beatrix, presentation held in 200 at the first Appenzeller Gesundheitskongress, Schwellbrunn, Switzerland

78 Further information: Lee, Dr. John R.: The American gynaecologist published articles on fluoride in The Journal of the Canadian Dental Association, volume 53, 1987, p. 763

et seq.; 'Review of Flouride: Benefits and Risks', U.S. Department of Health and Public Services, February 1991, p. 7, 31; 'The Truth about Mandatory Fluoridation', 15 April 1995

79 Gray, Dr., Allan S., director of the Division of Dental Health Services for British Colombia, Canada, Journal of the Canadian Dental Association, Vol. 10, p. 763–764

80 Colquhon, Dr., John, denstist and historian at the University of Oakland, New Zealand and head of the Oakland County Health Depatment

81 Dr. Phyllis Mullenix, Andover Massachusetts 01810-3347, P.O. Box 753. Dr. Mullenix is a researcher at various universities, such as the Toxicology Department at Forsyth Dental Center, Children's Hospital Medical Center in Boston

82 Clark, Dr., H. R., *Heilverfahren aller Krebsarten*, chapter Unnatürliche Chemikalien, pp. 122–126 [English original published under the title *The Cure for all Cancers*]

83 *Visionen 4/09, One Spirit Special*, pp. 25–27

84 Treben, Maria, *Gesundheit aus der Apotheke Gottes*, chapter Sauerklee [wood sorrel], p.44, 87 [English translation published under the title *Health through God's Pharmacy*]

85 ibid., chapter Schwedenkräuter [Swedish herbs], p. 61

86 ibid. chapter Vollbäder [full baths] , p. 8

87 Emoto, Masaru, *Wasserkristalle*

88 Detailed information on the healing water mentioned: Hürlimann, Gertrud, *Rute und Pendel*, chapter Lichtwässer, p. 236

89 E-mail: lourdes.water@lourdes-france.com

90 St. Leonhards Vertriebs GmbH, Mühlthalweg 54, Bad Leonhardspfunzen, 83071 Stephanskirchen, Germany

91 Strehlow, Dr., Wighard, *Die Ernährungstherapie der Hildegard von Bingen* 92 Strehlow, Dr., Wighard, *Hildegard-Heilkunde von A bis Z*

93 Strehlow, Dr., Wighard, *Die Edelsteinheilkunde der Hildegard von Bingen* 94 Further information: Hildegard Zentrum Bodensee, Strandweg 1, 78476 Allensbach, Germany. www.hildegardmed.com

95 Dr. Niedermaier Pharma GmbH, Taufkirchner Str. 59, 85662 Hohenbrunn, Germany. www.niedermaier-pharma.de

96 Blank, Dr. med., Karl-Heinz, Scheller, Ekkehard, Seidler, Johannes, Gans-windt, Thomas, Kohler, Dr. med., Axel, *»Damit müssen Sie jetzt leben!« NEIN Danke!*, information for therapists only

97 HOMÖOPATHIE-aktuell, Goethes Gespräch mit J. D. Falk, 25 Jan. 1813, 3/2005,

p. 9
98 Fintelmann, Prof. Dr. med., Volker, *Parkinson-Krankheit,* issue 207
99 Further information: Verein für anthroposophisch erweitertes Heilwesen e. V.,
Johannes-Kepler-Str. 56, 75378 Bad Liebenzell, Germnay
100 The German association for anthroposophic medicine, *Dachverband
Anthroposophische Medizin in Deutschland* (DAMiD), has a directory of anthroposophic
doctors and clinics: www.damid.de
101 Clark, Dr., H. R., *Heilverfahren aller Krebsarten,* chapter 1, pp. 28–43
[English original published under the title *The Cure for all Cancers*]
102 Frischknecht, Martin, *Gesundheit als Chance,* chap. Leberreinigung, pp. 138–139
103 Breuss, Rudolf, *Die Breuss Krebskur,* chap. Wichtige Tees zur Krebskur, p. 38 [English
translation published under the title *The Breuss Cancer Cure*]
104 Scheller, Ekkehard und Sabine, *Candidalismus?!*
105 Jentschura, Dr. h. c., Peter, Lohkämper, Josef, *Zivilisatoselos,* chap. Das
Wasserstoffperoxyd $H_2O_2$, pp. 75–87
106 See also www.aslan.info, Literature: Aslan, Prof. Dr., Ana, *The Effects of Gerovital H
Treatment in Parkinsonian Syndromes*
107 Krohne, Horst, *Handbuch für Heilende Hände,* chap. Parkinsonsche Krankheit, p.
100
108 Welt der Wunder, *Wie Musik das Gehirn heilt*, March 2008, pp. 14–23
109 Information on S.E.M. seminars for elementary meditation: Am Kreuzberg 9,
59955 Winterberg, Germany, www.elementare-meditation.de
110 Further information: Selbsthilfeorganisation *elementares Wissen e. V.,* Am
Kreuzberg 9, 59955 Winterberg, Germany, www.elementares-wissen.de
111 Clark, Dr., H. R., *Heilverfahren aller Krebsarten,* chap. Wie Sie sich testen, pp.
417–481 [English original published under the title *The Cure for all Cancers*]
112 Frischknecht, Martin, *Gesundheit als Chance,* chap. Grundlagen zur Anwendung, pp.
17–52
113 Karstädt, Uwe, *Entgiften statt vergiften,* chap. Powerquickzap, der Alleskönner, p.
230–231.
114 Frischknecht, Martin, *Gesundheit als Chance,* chap. Der QuickZap auf den
Philippinen, Dokumente zur Beurteilung des Leukämiefalles von JAM-JAM für
Fachleute. Der QuickZap in Mexiko, pp. 57–74
115 Kunhardt von, Gert, *kleiner aufwand grosse wirkung,* chap. Phänomenales

Ergebnis, p. 23–26

[116] Jentschura, Dr. h. c., Peter, Lohkämper, Josef, *Zivilisatoselos,* chap. Das Wasserstoffperoxyd $H_2O_2$, pp. 75–87

[117] Fliege, *Parkinson – Können Nadeln heilen,* December 2007, p. 64

[118] Inauris e. V., Esmarchstr. 26, 10407 Berlin, Germany, www.inauris.com/parkinson

[119] Deutsche Akademie für EDTA-Chelat Therapie e. V., www.chelat.biz

[120] Paturi, Felix R., *Indianische Heilpflanzen,* chap. Die Basis moderner Psychopharmaka, p. 71, 121

[121] ibid., chap. Zauberdrogen – Pflanzen der Götter, p. 94, chap. Anwendungen von A bis Z, p. 123

[122] Apotheken Umschau, *Heilende Tiergifte,* October 2007, pp. 62–67

[123] BIO, *Sanfte Medizin Lebenskunst Ernährung,* 5/2007, p. 34

[124] Schrott, Dr. med., Ernst, *Weihrauch,* chap. Wie wirkt Weihrauch in der Zelle, p. 70

[125] Welt der Wunder, *Wie Musik das Gehirn heilt,* March 2008, pp. 14–23

[126] Fliege, *Musik trainiert wichtige Gehirnfunktionen,* December 2009, p. 18

[127] a tempo 07/2007, *Parkinson, wenn die Bewegung aus dem Rhythmus gerät,* chap. Sprechstunde, p. 20/21, by Markus Sommer, www.gesund-heitaktiv-heilkunst.de

## Part III

1 Breuss, Rudolf, *Die Breuss Krebskur*, pp. 99–100 [English translation published under the title *The Breuss Cancer Cure*]

2 Frischknecht, Martin, *Gesundheit als Chance*, p. 204

3 Welt der Wunder, July 2010, p. 27

4 Karstädt, Uwe, *Entgiften statt vergiften*, p. 139

5 Welt der Wunder, April 2008, pp. 14–24

6 Karstädt, Uwe, *Entgiften statt vergiften*, p. 44

7 Welt der Wunder, September 2009, pp. 14–22

8 Jentschura, Dr. h. c., Peter, Lohkämper, Josef, *Zivilisatoselos*, p. 115

9 Elmadfa, Prof. Dr., Ibrahim, Muskat, Prof. Dr., E., Fritzsche, Dipl. oec. Troph., D., *E-Nummern*, pp. 12–72

10 Welt der Wunder, Sept. 2009, pp. 14–22

11 Jentschura, Dr. h. c., Peter, Lohkämper, Josef, *Zivilisatoselos*, p. 100, 123

12 Clark, Dr., H. R., *Heilverfahren aller Krebsarten*, p. 57 [English original published under the title *The Cure for all Cancers*]

13 Welt der Wunder, Sept. 2009, pp. 14–22

14 Welt der Wunder, June 2010, p. 91

15 Jentschura, Dr. h. c., Peter, Lohkämper, Josef, *Zivilisatoselos*, p. 120

16 Clark, Dr., H. R., *Heilverfahren aller Krebsarten*, p. 83, 89, 520 [English original published under the title *The Cure for all Cancers*]

17 Jentschura, Dr. h. c., Peter, Lohkämper, Josef, *Zivilisatoselos*, p. 116 et seq.

18 Karstädt, Uwe, *Entgiften statt vergiften*, p. 196, 198, 199

19 Elmadfa, Prof. Dr., Ibrahim, Muskat, Prof. Dr., E., Fritzsche, Dipl. oec. Troph., D., *E-Nummern*, pp. 12–72

20 Karstädt, Uwe, *Entgiften statt vergiften*, p. 162

21 ibid., p. 140

22 Welt der Wunder, Mai 2008, p. 48–49.

23 Scheller, Ekkehard und Sabine, *Candidalismus?!*, p. 55, pp. 74–88

24 Karstädt, Uwe, *Entgiften statt vergiften*, p. 11

25 Frischknecht, Martin, *Gesundheit als Chance*, p. 196, 198

26 Jentschura, Dr. h. c., Peter, Lohkämper, Josef, *Zivilisatoselos*, p. 24, pp. 125– 129

27 Karstädt, Uwe, *Entgiften statt vergiften*, p. 16, 58

28 Frischknecht, Martin, *Gesundheit als Chance*, p. 204

29 Karstädt, Uwe, *Entgiften statt vergiften*, p. 13, 23, 30, 42, 50

30 Scheller, Ekkehard und Sabine, *Candidalismus?!*, p. 74, 176
31 Jentschura, Dr. h. c., Peter, Lohkämper, Josef, *Zivilisatoselos*, p. 103 32 Welt der Wunder, Sept. 2009, pp. 14–22
33 Clark, Dr., H. R., *Heilverfahren aller Krebsarten*, p. 64 [English original published under the title *The Cure for all Cancers*]
34 ibid., p. 50, 94
35 Welt der Wunder, July 2007, pp. 12–21
36 Frischknecht, Martin, *Gesundheit als Chance*, p. 204
37 Jentschura, Dr. h. c., Peter, Lohkämper, Josef, *Zivilisatoselos*, p. 98, 102, 143
38 ibid., p. 82, 102–103., 136, 143
39 Scheller, Ekkehard und Sabine, *Candidalismus?!*, p. 120 40 Clark, Dr., H. R., *Heilverfahren aller Krebsarten*, p. 57 [English original published under the title *The Cure for all Cancers*]
41 Jentschura, Dr. h. c., Peter, Lohkämper, Josef, *Zivilisatoselos*, p. 136
42 Clark, Dr., H. R., *Heilverfahren aller Krebsarten*, p. 50, 57, 61–62, 64, 94, 104 et seq., 494 [English original published under the title *The Cure for all Cancers*]
43 Breuss, Rudolf, *Die Breuss Krebskur*, pp. 55–59, 98 [English translation published under the title *The Breuss Cancer Cure*]
44 Frischknecht, Martin, *Gesundheit als Chance*, p. 204
45 Karstädt, Uwe, *Entgiften statt vergiften*, p. 29, 47, 136
46 Scheller, Ekkehard und Sabine, *Candidalismus?!*, p. 140
47 Karstädt, Uwe, *Entgiften statt vergiften*, p. 42
48 Welt der Wunder, April 2008, pp. 14–22
49 Breuss, Rudolf, *Die Breuss Krebskur*, p. 101 [English translation published under the title *The Breuss Cancer Cure*]
50 Herbst, Erika, Die Lösung des Krebsproblems, Die Heilkunst von Morgen, pp. 123–140
51 Welt der Wunder, Sept. 2009, p. 14–22
52 Scheller, Ekkehard und Sabine, *Candidalismus?!*
53 Breuss, Rudolf, *Die Breuss Krebskur*, chap. Prostatakrebs/Hodenkrebs, p. 49 [English translation published under the title *The Breuss Cancer Cure*]
54 Clark, Dr., H. R., *Heilverfahren aller Krebsarten* [English original published under the title *The Cure for all Cancers*]
55 Frischknecht, Martin, *Gesundheit als Chance*
56 Jentschura, Dr. h. c., Peter, Lohkämper, Josef, *Zivilisatoselos*
57 Kellenberger, Richard und Kopsche, Friedrich, *Mineralstoffe nach Dr. Schüßler*
58 Jentschura, Dr.h.c., Peter, Lohkämper, Josef, *Zivilisatoselos*
59 Breuss, Rudolf, *Die Breuss Krebskur* [English translation published under the title *The Breuss Cancer Cure*]

# References


Arntz, William, Betsy Chasse, Mark Vicente, *Bleep*, Vak-Verlag, Kirchzarten

Bach, Dr, Edward, *Heile Dich selbst mit Bachblüten*, Knaur MensSana, Munich, 1st German edition, 2000

Bakalayan, Alan E., *Sanftes Heilen mit Bio-Frequenzen*, Michels-Verlag

Bakalayan, Alan E., *Parasiten – die verborgene Ursache vieler Erkrankungen*, Goldmann Verlag, Munich

Bartens, Dr. med., Werner, *Das Ärztehasserbuch, Ein Insider packt aus*, Knaur-Verlag, Munich, 2007

Blank, Dr. med. Karl-Heinz, Scheller Ekkehard, Seidler Johannes, Ganswindt Thomas, Kohler, Dr. med. Axel, *»Damit müssen Sie jetzt leben!« NEIN Danke!*, Teamdruck Verlag, Weyhe, 2008

Blüchel, Kurt G., *Heilen verboten – Töten erlaubt*, Goldmann Verlag, München, 2nd edition, paperback edition, 2004

Bollhalder, Johannes, *Die Quelle zum Heilwerden, Ganzheit – Lebensgefühl – Quantensprung*, Lebensquell Verlag, Luzern, 2005

Bösch, Dr. med., PD., Jakob, *Versöhnen und Heilen, Spiritualität, Wissenschaft und Wirtschaft im Einklang*, AT Verlag, Baden and Munich, 2008

Bösch, Dr. med., PD., Jakob, *Spirituelles Heilen und Schulmedizin*, AT Verlag, Baden and Munich, 2008

Brandes, Vera/Salvesen, Christian, *Die heilende Kraft der Klänge, Schwingungen und Gefühle*, O. W. Barth Verlag, Frankfurt

Breuss, Rudolf, *Krebs/Leukämie*, Eigenverlag Rudolf Breuss, Nüziders, new edition 2005

Carson, Rolf, *Zukunftschance Gesundheit*, Günther Albert Ulmer Verlag, 1st edition, 2007

Ciccolo, Enza Maria, *Lichtwässer, Wasser der heilenden Liebe*, AT-Verlag, Baden and Munich

Clark, Dr., Hulda, *Die Heilung aller Krebsarten*, New Century Press, Chula Vista, USA, 2004 [English original published under the title *The Cure for all Cancers*]

Dunkenberger, Thomas, *Das tibetische Heilbuch*, Windpferd Verlag, Aitrang, 2nd edition, 2002

Elmadfa, Prof. Dr., Ibrahim, Muskat, Prof. Dr., E., Fritzsche, Dipl. oec. Troph., D., *ENummern*, GU-Verlag, Munich, updated edition, 1996

Emoto, Masaru, *Wasserkristalle,* KOHA-Verlag, Burgrain, no date [English translations of some of Emoto's works also available]

Feldenkrais, Moshé, *Abenteuer im Dschungel des Gehirns – Der Fall Doris,* Suhrkamp Verlag, Berlin, Taschenbuch 663, 1st edition, 1981

Fintelmann, Prof. Dr. med., Volker, *Parkinson-Krankheit, Wege zur aktiven Begegnung,* issue 207, 2003, Anthrosana/Verein für anthroposophisch erweitertes Heilwesen e. V., Johannes-Kepler-Str. 56, 75378 Bad Liebenzell

Fleig, Harald, *Heilen über die Wirbelsäule nach Breuss – Dorn – Fleig,* Verlag B. u. H. Fleig, Wehr, volumes 1 & 2, 4th edition, 2008

Frischknecht, Martin, *Gesundheit als Chance,* Günther Albert Ulmer Verlag, Tuningen

Grün, Siegrid, Neidhardt, Jan, *ARONIA Unentdeckte Heilpflanze,* Edition buntehunde, abridged version, 2010

Heepen, Günther H., *Schüssler-Salze typgerecht,* GU-Verlag, Munich, 1st edition, 2007

Heller, Diane Pool/ Heller, Laurence S., *Crash-Kurs zur Selbsthilfe nach Verkehrsunfällen,* Synthesis-Verlag, Essen

Herbst, Erika, *Lösung des Krebsproblems, Die Heilkunst von Morgen, Andere Hilfen und Tabus,* Selbsthilfegruppe Mündige Bürger, self-published, 3rd edition, 2006

Hering, Dr. med., Constantin/Haehl, Dr. med., Richard, *Homöopathischer Hausarzt,* Frommann-Holzboog Verlag (G.Hauff), Stuttgart, 1908

Hürlimann, Gertrud I., *Rute und Pendel, Ein methodisch aufgebautes Lehrbuch für Einsteiger und Fortgeschrittene,* Oesch Verlag, Zurich, 11th edition 2005

Hüther, Dr. med., Harald, *Spezialratgeber Ernährung, Vitalstoffe & Gesundheit* Institut Opti-Mahl, Tiefenbach

Jahr, Dr. med., *Homöopathischer Leitfaden,* Verlag für homöopathische Literatur, Hamburg 2003, reprint of 1869 edition

Jänke, Lutz, *Macht Musik schlau,* Verlag Hans Huber, Bern Jentschura, Peter, Dr. h. c., Lohkämper, Josef, *Zivilisatoselos,* Verlag Peter Jentschura, Münster, 2nd extended edition, 2005

Jentschura, Dr. h. c., Peter, Lohkämper, Josef, *Gesundheit durch Entschlackung*, Verlag Peter Jentschura, Münster, 14th edition, 2006

Kalbermatten, Roger und Hildegard, *Pflanzliche Urtinkturen-Wesen und Anwendung*, AT-Verlag, Baden and Munich, 2007

Karstädt, Uwe, *Entgiften statt vergiften*, TAS Distribution Ltd., London, updated edition, 2009

Karstädt, Uwe, *Die 7 Revolutionen der Medizin,* TAS Customertimes Ltd., London

Kellenberger, Richard, Kopsche, Friedrich, *Mineralstoffe nach Dr. Schüssler,* AT Verlag, Baden

Knophius, Heike, *Säure-Basen-Balance,* GU-Verlag, Munich, 7th edition, 2007

Krebs, Harald, *Die Praxis der Vitamin C Hochdosis-Therapie,* Verlag Medizin und Management, Hamm

Krohne, Horst, *Handbuch für Heilende Hände, Das A–Z der Übertragung von Heilenergie,* Ansata Verlag, Munich, 10th edition, 2007

Kuby, Clemens, *Unterwegs in die nächste Dimension,* Kösel-Verlag, Munich, 12th edition, 2006

Kuby, Clemens, *Heilung das Wunder in uns, Selbstheilungsprozesse entdecken,* Kösel-Verlag, Munich, 6th edition, 2007

Kühni, Werner/Walter von Holst, *Taschenlexikon der Heilsteine,* AT-Verlag Baden and Munich, 3rd edition, 2006

Kunhardt von, Gert, *kleiner aufwand grosse wirkung, Phänomen Trampolin,* Verlag Bellicon Deutschland, Cologne, 11th edition, 2010

Lad, Vasant, *Das Ayurveda Heilbuch,* Edition Schangrila, Haldenwang, 2nd edition, 1987

Langen, Prof. Dr. med., Dietrich, *Autogenes Training,* GU-Verlag, Munich, 7th edition, 2004

Liem, Torsten/Tsoldimos, Christine, *Osteopathie, Die sanfte Lösung bei Blockaden* Ariston Verlag, Munich

Lipton, Bruce, *Intelligente Zellen: Wie Erfahrungen unsere Gene steuern,* Koha-Verlag, Burgrain [English original published under the title *The Wisdom of Your Cells: How Your Beliefs Control Your Biology*]

Lorber, Jakob, *Die Heilkraft des Sonnenlichts,* Lorber-Verlag und Turmverlag, Bietigheim [English translation published under the title

*The Healing Power of Sunlight*]
Maar, Prof. Dr., Klaus, *Rebell gegen den Krebs,* Kopp Verlag, Rottenburg
Neukirchen, Heide, *HEXAL-Kapitalismus – Der Aufstieg der Brüder Strüngmann,* Campus-Verlag, Frankfurt
Panos, Dr. med., M.B./Heimlich, Jane, *Homöopatische Hausapotheke,* Heyne-Verlag, Dresden, 2002
Paturi, Felix R., *Indianische Heilpflanzen, Mit heimischen und exotischen Pflanzen nach der indianischen Heiltradition Krankheiten vorbeugen und behandeln,* G. Reichel Verlag, Weilersbach, 2007
Phatak, *Homöopathische Arzneimittellehre,* Urban & Fischer, Munich, 2004
Pschyrembel, *Klinisches Wörterbuch,* Walter de Gruyter Verlag, Berlin, 260th revised edition, 2004
Pschyrembel, *Naturheilkunde und alternative Heilverfahren,* Walter de Gruyter Verlag, Berlin, 3rd completely revised edition, 2006
Pschyrembel, *Therapeutisches Wörterbuch,* Walter de Gruyter Verlag, Berlin, 2nd revised and expanded edition 2001
Raslan, Gamal, *Der sanfte Weg zur Mitte: Die Dorn-Methode,* Aurum Verlag/Kamphausen Verlag, Bielefeld, 5th edition, 2007
Richter, Isolde, *Lehrbuch für Heilpraktiker,* Urban & Fischer, Munich, 2000
Scheffer, Mechthild, *Bach-Blütentherapie – Theorie und Praxis,* Hugendubel Verlag, Munich
Schramm, Georg, *Lassen Sie es mich mal so sagen …* Blessing Verlag, Munich, 1st edition, 2007
Schrott, Dr. med., Ernst, *Weihrauch – Seine außergewöhnliche Wirkung neu entdeckt,* Aurum Verlag/Kamphausen Verlag, Munich, 2nd edition, 2004
Scheller, Ekkehard und Sabine, *Candidalismus?!, Candida-Pilze & Parasiten in unserem Blut, die schleichende Gefahr! Heilung durch ein harmonisches Blutmilieu,* Ulmer Verlag, Tuningen, 2nd edition, 2007
Sha, Sonia, *Am Menschen getestet,* Redline-Wirtschaftsverlag, Munich
Sharamon, Shalila/Baginski, Bodo, *Die Schisandra-Beere,* Windpferd-Verlag, Oberstdorf, 1st edition, 2009
Sharamom, Shalaila, Baginski, Bodo J., *Goji – die ultimative Superfrucht,* Windpferd Verlag, Oberstdorf, 5th edition 2009
Shioya, Dr., Nobuo, *Der Jungbrunnen des Dr. Shioya,* KOHA-Verlag,

Burgrain, 4th edition, 2009

Silber, Otto-Heinrich, *Klangtherapie – Wege zur inneren Harmonie,* Traumzeit-Verlag, Battweiler

Spalding, Baird T., *Leben und Lehren der Meister im fernen Osten Band 4–5,* Schirner Verlag, Darmstadt, 1st edition, 2004

Strehlow, Dr., Wighard, *Die Edelsteinheilkunde der Hildegard von Bingen,* Weltbild-Verlag, Augsburg, 2008

Tag, Karin, *Mysterium Kristallschädel,* Heyne-Verlag, Dresden, 2009

Thurman, Robert A. F., *Das tibetische Totenbuch,* special edition, Fischer TB Verlag, Frankfurt am Main, 2000

Treben, Maria, *Gesundheit aus der Apotheke Gottes,* Ennsthaler Verlag, A-Steyr, 87th edition, 2007 [English translation published under the title *Health through God's Pharmacy*]

Upledger, Dr., John E., *Auf den inneren Arzt hören,* Allegria im Ullstein Taschenbuch-Verlag, Berlin, 2nd edition, 2007 [English original published under the title *Your inner physician and you*]

alla Via, Gudrun, *Lichtwässer und ihre verborgenen Heilkräfte,* AT-Verlag, Baden and Munich

Virapen, John, *Nebenwirkung TOD,* Neuer Europa Verlag, Leipzig, 3rd edition, 2008 [English original published under the title *Side Effects: Death*]

Wagner, Dr. med., Franz, *Akupressur,* GU-Verlag, Munich, 2003 Werner, Michael, Dr. med./Stöckli, Thomas/Bösch, PD. Dr. med., J., *Leben durch Lichtnahrung,* AT Verlag, Baden and Munich, 2005 Yoda, Prof., Dr., Peter., *Ein medizinischer Insider packt aus,* Sensei-Verlag, Kernen, 2008

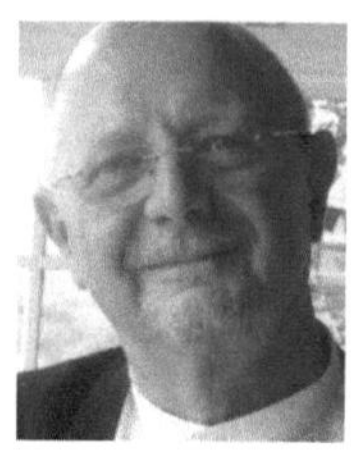 The author Manfred J.Poggel

Beginning in early childhood, the author suffered from rheumatic diseases, chronic polyarthritis, sclerosis, Osgood-Schlatter disease and other diseases, which nowadays are characterised as fibromyalgia. He therefore had to learn to deal with these diagnoses at an early age, to ignore them when he could and to lead a busy and fulfilling life in spite of them.

Today it is clear to him that his body was damaged early on due to poor nutrition, poor living conditions and the desperate situations during the Second World War and post-war years.

From 2002 onwards, his Parkinson's disease became so severe that by 2003 he was no longer able to work. The dreaded diagnosis of Parkinson's disease was officially confirmed in 2004 and legally recognised by a court in 2006.

After several key experiences, he began his search for effective healing at the end of 2006. After phasing out the use of chemical medications, various connections between causes and effects became clear.

He received information on the incredible possibilities that natural medicine had to offer for treating his disease. He recorded and checked all of the tips he was given and evaluated them for himself. It was a difficult process. It was not easy to choose the therapies that were right for him.

Nevertheless, he dared to try them because he always, always had the feeling that he was being guided and that he would become healthy again. He experienced the first small successes in 2009.

He felt how he was gradually getting better. In autumn 2010, he was finally able to stop using his natural therapies.

Today he can say that he is healed.

He has overcome not only the 'incurable' Parkinson's disease but also all other illnesses from earlier in his life. Over these years he learnt to change his lifestyle and diet and to help people change their perspective.
He passes on his experiences and findings to all members in his independent charitable self-help organisation, *Selbsthilfeorganisation elementares Wissen e. V.*   www.elementares-wissen.de

## Von dem Autor ebenfalls erschienen

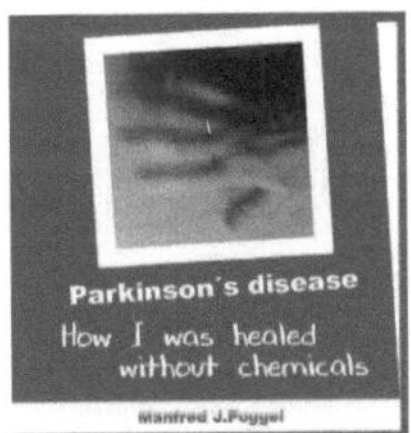


**Printausgabe - Parkinson´s disease - ISBN 978-620-3-57568-2**
**Ebook - Parkinson´s disease - ISBN 978-3-9819844-6-0**

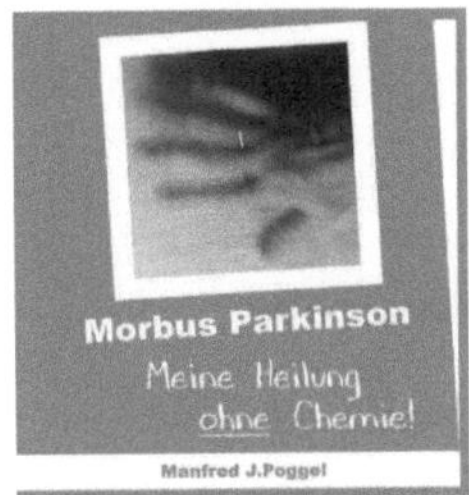


**Morbus Parkinson – Meine Heilung ohne Chemie**

368 Seiten - **ISBN 978-3-9819844-4-6**

Parkinson ist heilbar! Das klingt unglaublich? Manfred J. Poggel weiß, wovon er spricht. Er selbst hatte diese Krankheit in einem fortgeschrittenen Stadium. Da ihm die Schulmedizin keine Aussicht auf Heilung bot, fing er an, nach den Ursachen der Krankheit zu forschen und alternative Heilmethoden zu ergründen. Er begann ein neues Leben *ohne* Gifte.

In seinem sehr persönlichen Gesundheitsratgeber lässt Manfred J. Poggel den Leser teilhaben an seinen Erfahrungen mit über 30 Therapieformen.

Er gibt keine Heilungversprechen, sondern er beschreibt seinen ganz eigenen Weg zur Genesung, der über Ansätze wie Entsäuerung, Meditation, Akupunktur, Homöopathie und vieles mehr führte.

Sein zentrales Anliegen ist es, Wege der Früherkennung und der Prophylaxe aufzuzeigen.

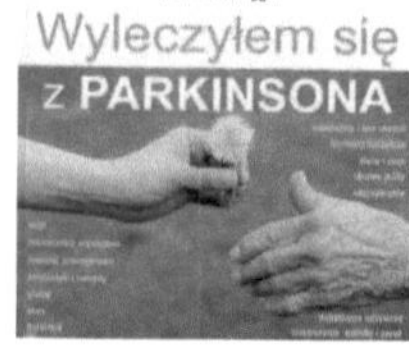


**polnische Ausgabe bei amazon als Printausgabe**

**ISBN-10: 8376491415   ISBN-13: 978-837641417**  -  KOS-Verlag

Parkinson jest uleczalny!

Brzmi nieprawdopodobnie? Manfred J. Poggel wie, o czym mówi. Sam mial zaawansowana forme parkinsona. Poniewaz medycyna akademicka nie byla w stanie zaoferowac mu powrotu do zdrowia, sam zaczal szukac przyczyny choroby i badac je oraz wypróbowal na sobie alternatywne metody leczenia. W ten sposób rozpoczal nowe zycie bez toksyn.

Drzenie nie oznacza parkinsona!

Wielu ludzi nie zdaje sobie z tego sprawy: drzenie oraz inne objawy choroby parkinsona towarzysza nie tylko chorobie parkinsona, ale również chorobom jej podobnym, takim jak syndrom niespokojnych nóg czy stwardnienie rozsiane. Wszystkie te schorzenia maja wspólny mianownik - ich przyczyna lezy w jelitach.

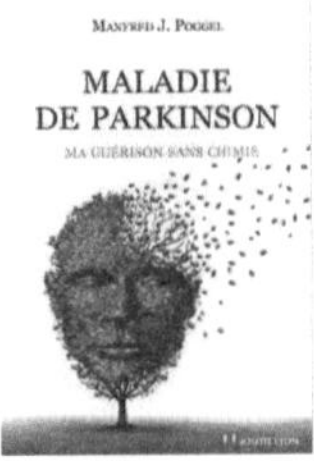

**Brosché et Format Kindle, Editeur: Josette Lyon**

**ISBN-10: 2843193524   ISBN-13: 978-2843193521**

**amazon.fr**  Maladie de Parkinson-Ma guerison sans chimie
https://www.amazon.fr/gp/product/B014USGET8/ref=s9_simh_gw_g351_i1_r?pf_rd_m=A1X6FK5RDHNB96&pf_rd
_s=desktop-&pf_rd_r=D1N5S8H901FTYDVQQBZJ&pf_rd_t=36701&pf_rd_p=ea4deef1-7693-4901-adb4-
00b9fcea23bf&pf_rd_i=desktop

Cela paraît incroyable ? Manfred J. Poggel sait de quoi il parle. Il souffrait lui-même de cette maladie à un stade avancé. La médecine traditionnelle ne lui offrant aucune perspective de guérison, il se mit à chercher les causes de la maladie et à explorer des méthodes thérapeutiques alternatives. Il commença une vie nouvelle sans chimie. Depuis deux ans, il est considéré comme guéri — et même ses nombreuses pathologies préexistantes ont disparu. L'auteur présente les 30 formes de thérapies différentes qui lui ont permis de guérir. Il ne fait aucune promesse, mais décrit son chemin de guérison tout à fait personnel, qui le conduisit vers de nouvelles approches thérapeutiques : la désacidification, la méditation, l'acupuncture, l'homéopathie, l'ayurvéda, l'argent colloïdal, le yoga, la cure Breuss, et bien d'autres. Sa principale préoccupation consiste à suggérer de nouvelles pistes permettant le dépistage précoce de la maladie de Parkinson. Grâce à des conseils avisés et à de nombreuses fiches pratiques, il montre la voie à tous ceux qui sont disposés à s'ouvrir à de nouveaux schémas de pensée et qui font le choix d'une guérison sans chimie.

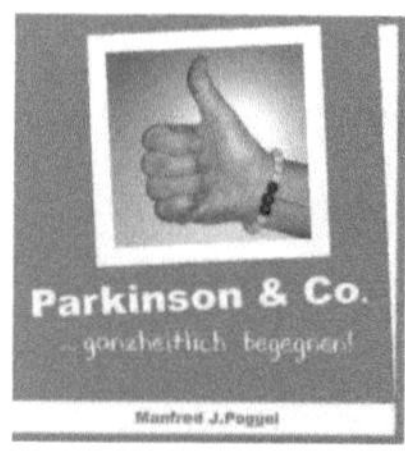


**NEU** in 2018

**1. Auflage als Print ISBN: 978-3-9819844-2-2**
   **eBook ISBN: 978-3-9819844-1-5**

**Eigenverlag  S.E.M. Renate Poggel-Zündorf, Manfred J.Poggel**

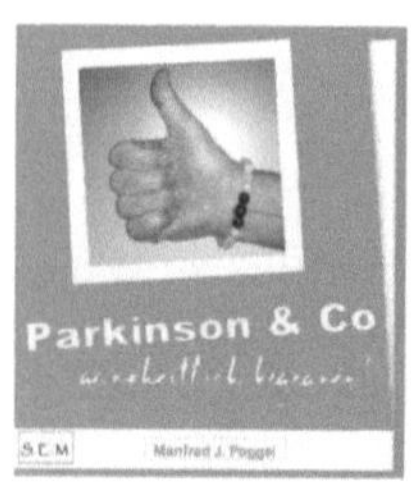


# Nouveau en 2018

**eBook et Format Kindle  ISBN: 978-3-9819844-3-9**
**Editeur:  S.E.M. Renate Poggel-Zündorf, Manfred J.Poggel**

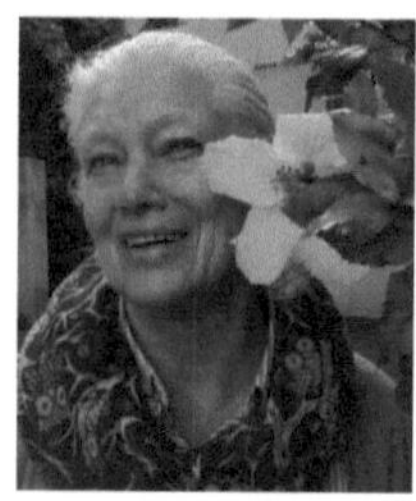

**Verlegerin und Autorin Renate Poggel-Zündorf**

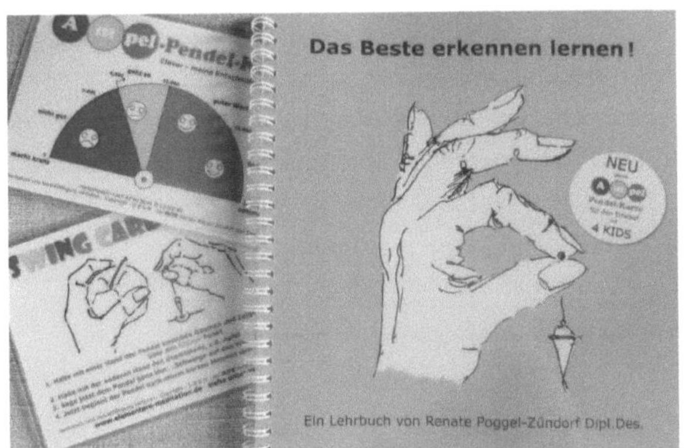


**Das Radiästhesie-Lehrbuch** : Das Beste erkennen lernen !

**ISBN: 978-3-00-042878-4**

**Mein Pendel ist ein Werkzeug und unterstützt meine täglichen Entscheidungen**

In den neuesten Ergebnissen der Biophysik ist es möglich die allgegenwärtigen vorhandenen Schwingungen unseres täglichen Lebens zu messen und endlich zu beweisen. Die Mystifizierung des Pendels ist damit endgültig vorbei.

Im Alltag zeigt mir mein Pendel das optimale "Wie und Was" für mich und meine Familie. Aus dieser Erfahrung werden hier mit völlig neuartigen Tabellen und Diagrammen viele praxisbezogene Anwendungsmöglichkeiten leicht verständlich vermittelt. Speziell auf die Bereiche der vielfältigen Ernährungsangebote und der Körperpflege, dem Wohlbefinden und Wohlgefühl für die Wohnung und den Arbeitsplatz wird hier ausführlich eingegangen.

*Als Besonderheit und **absoluter Neuheit** gibt es herausnehmbare Pendelkarten in den Ampelfarben*, die auf den ersten Blick erkennen lassen, ob das gewählte Produkt meinen Anforderungen entspricht. Die Devise: vor Ort schon Fehlkäufe vermeiden, nur Artikel mit hohen Schwingungen auswählen; denn das Wohl meiner Familie hat Priorität.

In jeder Familie sollte wenigstens ein Mitglied pendeln können.

**Beginne jetzt!** **"Das Bessere vom Guten zu unterscheiden"**

**Bestellungen für alle deutschsprachigen Ausgaben:**

**www.sem-verlag.de**

www.elementares-wissen.de/Bücher
www.elementare-meditation.de
www.amazon.de

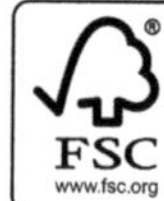